Herbs & Liver Health

A herbal medicine pocket guide

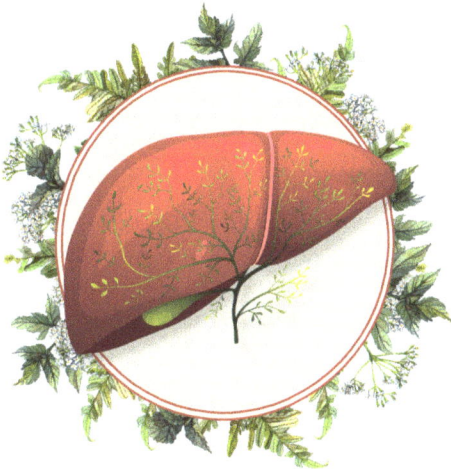

Sarah Murphy

ND. Dip. Herb URHP

Herbs & Liver Health: A Herbal Medicine Pocket Guide

© 2020 Sarah Murphy

The moral rights of the author have been asserted.

The information contained in this book is presented for interest only. Neither Herbary Books nor the author accept any liability relating to the use of this information. Please consult your medical herbalist or physician if you are unsure about following any of the advice in this book.

ISBN 978-1-9163396-6-8

HERBARYBOOKS

Published by Herbary Books
Caernarfon, Wales
www.herbarybooks.com
contact@herbarybooks.com

Content

This book is designed to serve as a 'pocket guide' to liver health through the use of nurturing herbal remedies and healing foods. The advice which follows is based on my own personal experience of using plant medicines in a clinical setting over the last twelve years. I hope you'll find it to be a practical (but most of all, useful) guide. The goal is to inspire you to learn more about herbs and how to use them effectively, as well as introduce you to some novel ways of incorporating them into your daily life.

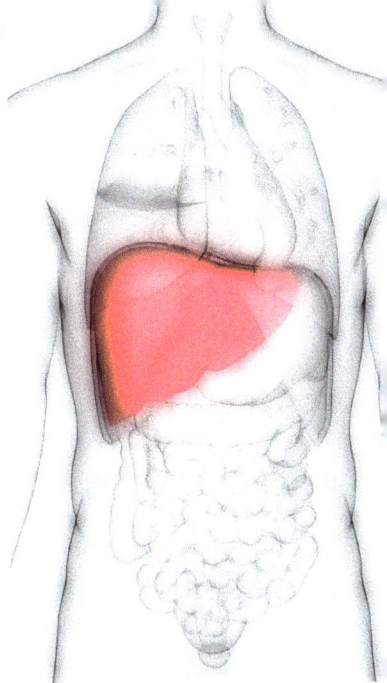

The plants described in this book can be easily sourced from your grocery store or grown at home. Most can also be found growing abundantly in the wild, or of course obtained from your local herbalist.

Please be aware that the information contained in these pages is intended to serve as an educational resource, and is not designed to replace the advice of your physician or medical health care practitioner. The author and publishers accept no liability for any claims which might arise from the use of any remedy or strategy described in this book.

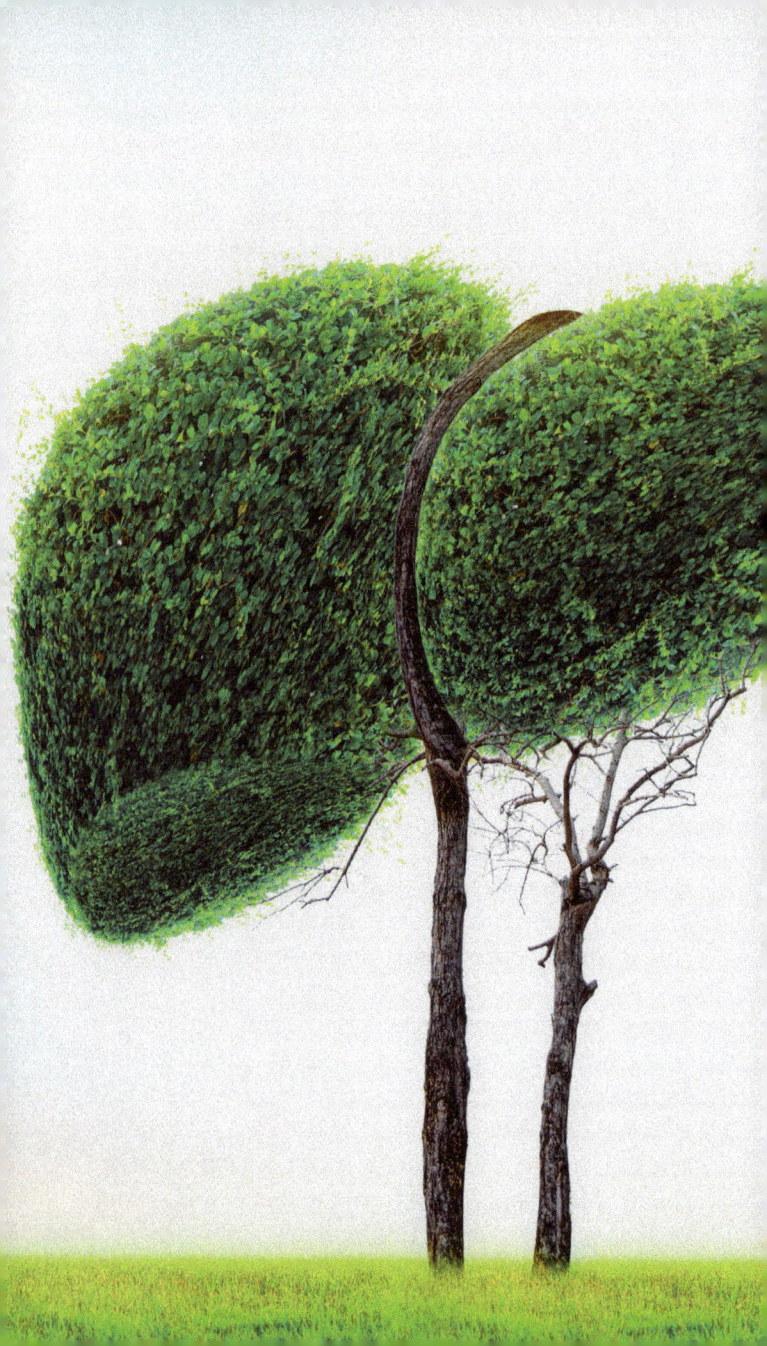

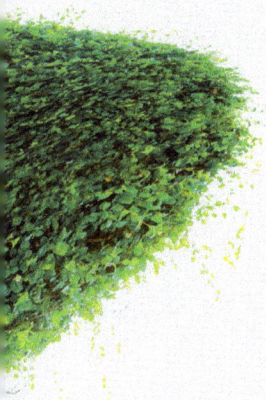

INTRODUCTION

Your amazing liver

The liver is one of the hardest working organs in the body. It is responsible for more than five hundred vital functions (that we know of), and probably many more besides. A big chemical company would have to build acres of plant to carry out anywhere near the amount of work this three pound organ does on a daily basis.

Yet unlike other organs such as the bladder, heart, or stomach, we hardly give it a second thought. It steadfastly goes about the day performing innumerable incredible feats; any one of which were to go wrong would quickly turn into a medical emergency.

Things like:

- Removing bacteria, drug residues and alcohol from the bloodstream
- Storing essential minerals such as iron
- Producing the bile needed by the digestive system to break down fats
- Manufacturing important immune enhancing substances
- Metabolising protein and carbohydrates to provide cells with energy
- Helping to keep hormone levels in balance
- Processing nutrients absorbed by the intestines
- Making essential chemicals that help blood clot properly
- Producing up to four litres of digestive fluids each and every day

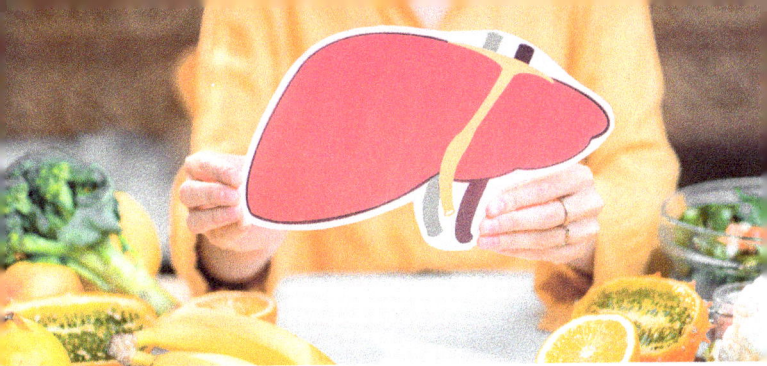

Your liver has an enormous amount of reserves and a huge capacity for regeneration. Disease can destroy as much as 85% of its working cells and it will still continue to dutifully carry out its jobs. As much as 80% can be cut away in surgery and it will still continue to function. It can also do something that other organs can't do - it has the remarkable ability to rebuild itself and repair the damage.

On top of all the tasks on your liver's 'to do' list, it also has the unenviable responsibility of defending you from the toxic effects of the modern world, protecting you from things like:

- Air pollution from traffic and smog
- Chemicals contained in hygiene products
- Additives in the food and beverages you consume
- Toxic coatings on kitchen utensils and surfaces
- Chemicals in your home and office furnishings

The list of pollutants and chemical substances it has to contend with goes on and on.

Despite its far reaching influence across numerous bodily systems, many people are unaware just how much their health issues could be improved, if only they paid more attention to their liver.

Common signs and symptoms of a poorly functioning liver

The liver is sometimes described as a silent organ, yet in times of trouble it has ways of showing you it is under stress. Although some of these signs are urgent enough to indicate a speedy visit to the doctor, many are subtle grumbles of complaint designed to make you sit up and take note that something is in need of attention.

Listed below are some of the most common signs your liver might be functioning below par.

- Painful or absent periods
- Chronic fatigue and lethargy
- Excessive sweating
- Bruising easily
- Difficulty digesting fats
- An inability to lose weight
- Problems with elimination via the bowels
- Anxiety or depression (liver qi stagnation)

Interestingly, the eyes are also closely linked to your liver function. They can provide clear clues when urgent attention is needed.

For example:

- If someone develops hepatitis, the whites of their eyes turn yellow
- People with hyperthyroidism (hormone regulation) often have bulging eyes
- Redness under the eyes can be a sign of anaemia (the liver stores iron)

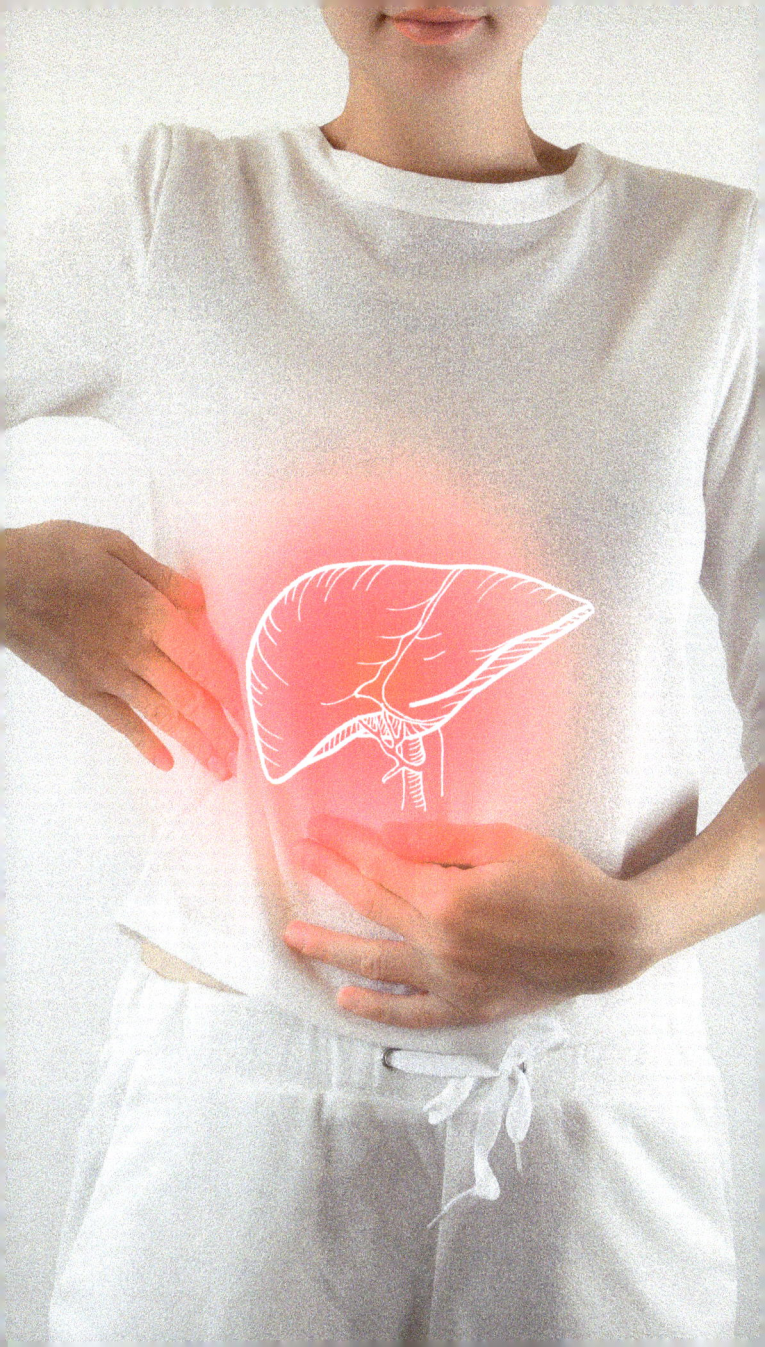

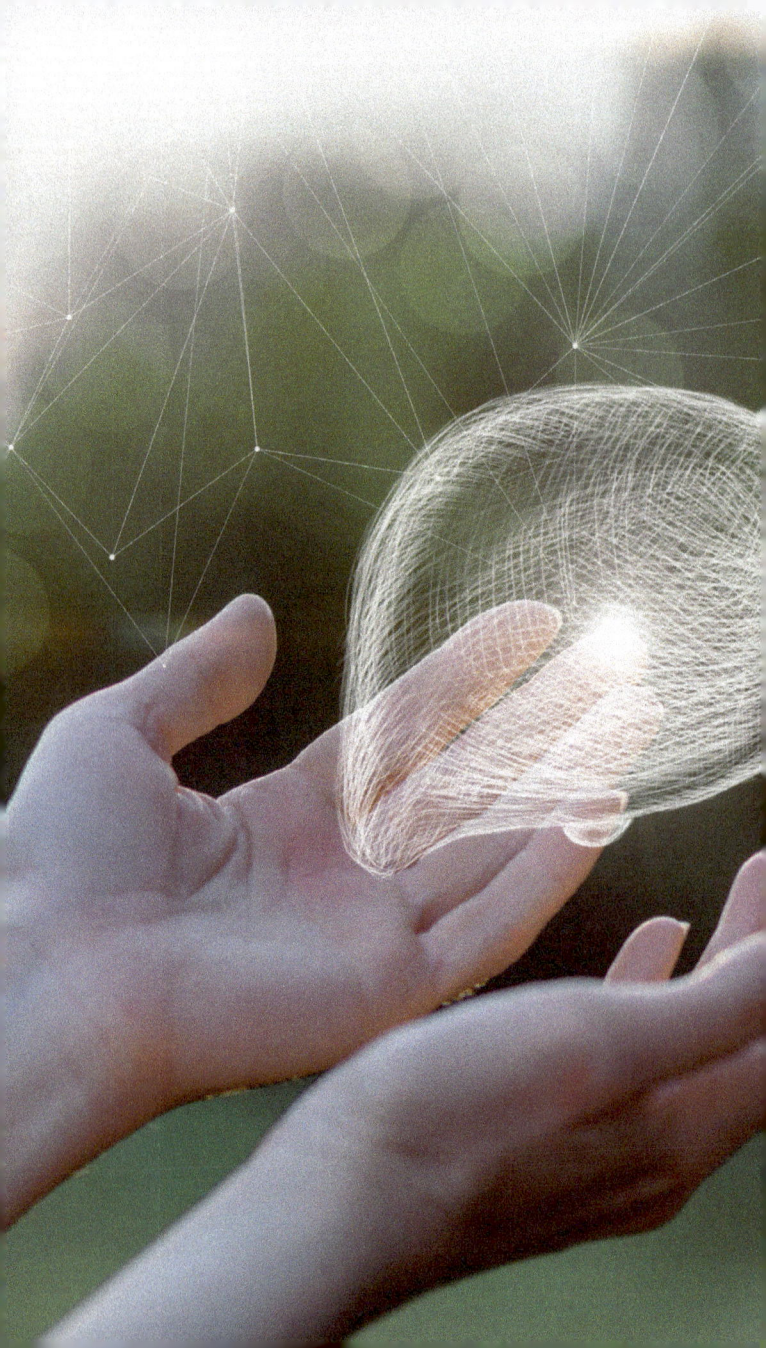

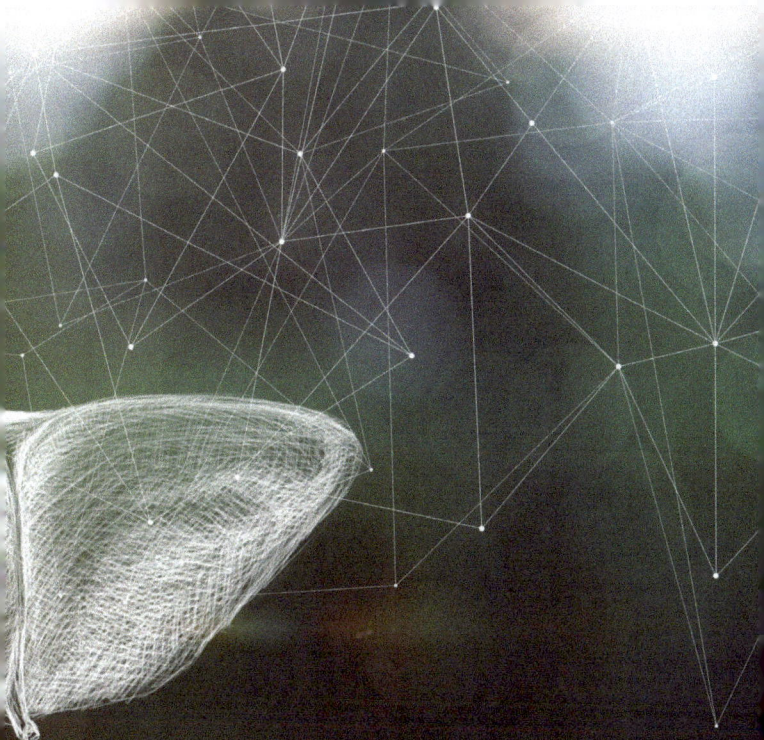

What does your liver actually do?

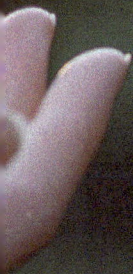

As this book is not intended to be a medical text on anatomy and physiology, only a brief overview of the main functions of the liver is provided. The purpose of this short explanation is to enable you to gain a better understanding of how herbs can be used to support this amazing organ on a practical level.

The liver to gastro-intestinal (GI) pathway

As you may already know, the liver plays a vital role in the proper functioning of your digestive system. One of its main jobs is to produce bile, a fluid whose purpose is to break down fat from the food you eat.

Cells called hepatocytes make up about 55 - 65% percent of your liver's mass. These cells secrete bile, which then passes to the gallbladder where the thin watery liquid is collected and reduced down into a very concentrated form. Every time you eat food, bile moves from your gallbladder into the duodenum (the first section of your small intestine, the bit which receives partially digested food from your stomach.)

Put very simply, this is then broken down into:

- Nutrients which are delivered back to your cells, tissues and organs
- Waste material which is either expelled by the bowel (fat soluble toxins are excreted in stools) or kidneys (water soluble toxins are eliminated via urine, or through the skin as sweat.)

The GI to liver pathway

Nutrients and waste products created from the food you eat are absorbed from your digestive tract and through the gut wall. At this point they enter into the portal vein. Imagine this as being a bit like 'dirty blood' which is returned to the liver ready to be metabolised, processed and shipped out again in the form of fresh nutrients for cells, or expelled as waste products as described above.

In short, your liver is a very efficient <u>blood purification plant</u>. A properly functioning liver that's not overwhelmed by its duties is much better able to help rid your body of toxic waste. This means you're less likely to succumb to food allergies, colds and flu, lethargy, depression and a myriad of other ailments that a large percentage of the population put up with on a daily basis.

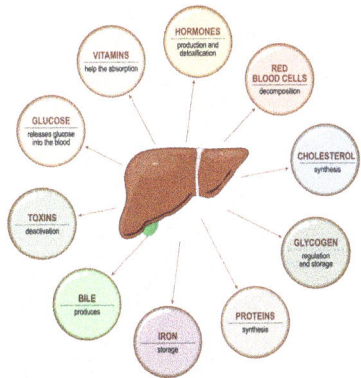

The liver to the rest of your body

After the huge clean up job your liver neatly performs, nutrients from this freshly 'purified blood' are then distributed to cells, tissues and organs throughout your body. The cells take up the nutrients and the whole wonderful cycle begins again.

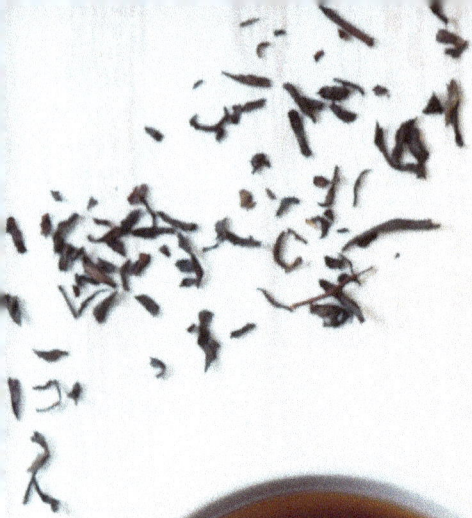

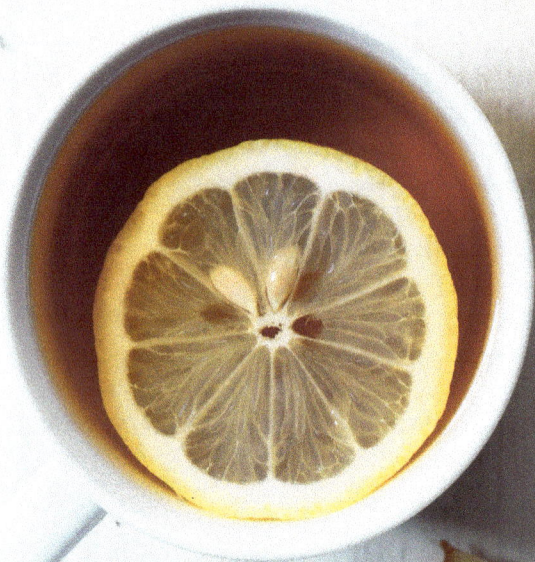

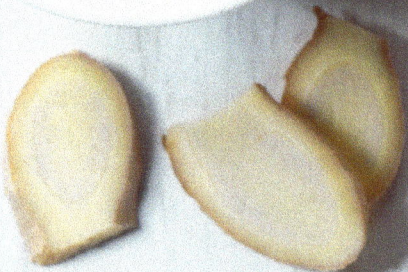

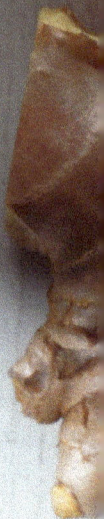

The liver & detoxification

If you were fortunate enough to live in a stress free world where you were able to breathe fresh air, and have unlimited access to vibrant, life giving foods, your liver could dutifully carry out its daily tasks with hardly any problems at all. However, we all know that this is far from reality.

Increased consumption of processed foods and exposure to stress and environmental toxins mean these processes and pathways are commonly impaired. Despite this, many allopathic practitioners (and most of the general public at large) continue to labour under the impression that cleansing or detoxifying the liver is a pointless waste of time.

It's clear from what we've already discussed, that if your liver wasn't on a relentless mission to detoxify then the inevitable result would be death. Of course this is absolutely true, but the fact remains that life in the modern age puts a huge amount of pressure on your liver to keep up. It can easily become overwhelmed. Relieving it of some of its burdens and allowing it a bit more time to catch up with its jobs can be very beneficial.

Let's compare this to an example we're all familiar with – cleaning the house:

Every day you do household chores; washing the dishes, vacuuming the carpets, wiping down surfaces, washing the dishes etc etc etc... There are many jobs that need to be done on a daily basis in order to simply 'keep on top of things.' In reality, most people lead busy lives, and don't have the time to do a deep clean every single day. However, you can only go on like this for so long until the little jobs you never get around to start to niggle. The guttering may need attention, the cupboard under the sink may start looking grimy, and spiders may begin to make a home for themselves on the tops of neglected dusty shelves. Inevitably there comes a point where you feel the urge to throw open the windows and have a really good spring clean.

We can apply this same analogy to the liver.

As Simon Mills succinctly explains in his Essential Book of Herbal Medicine.

> *"The toxicity thesis of disease proposes the sensible hypothesis that the removal of waste materials from the body is absolutely essential for good health.*
> *Several eliminatory functions share the task (of removing waste from the system) failure or suppression of one will lead to extra burdens and possible signs of distress in others, and will have potentially widespread implications for general health."*

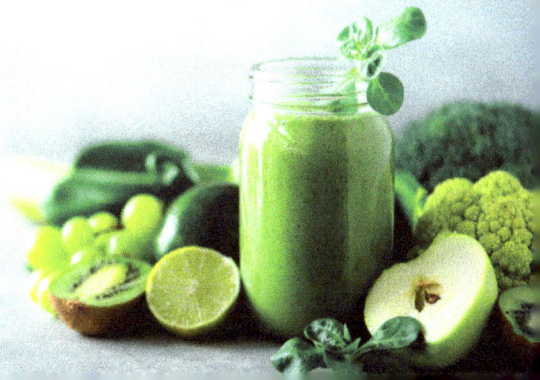

Sluggish liver function has far reaching effects felt by the entire body. A helping hand in the form of herbs, and making small dietary or lifestyle changes, can make a huge difference to the daily functioning of this very important organ, and of course, your overall health.

Liver function can be impaired in a number of ways which have a direct impact on your wellbeing.

For example:

• A lack of bile production means that food isn't broken down properly. This leads to poor elimination and stagnant material building up in the bowel. Once this pathway becomes impaired, health issues such as constipation, leaky gut, lethargy and even some autoimmune conditions can be the result.

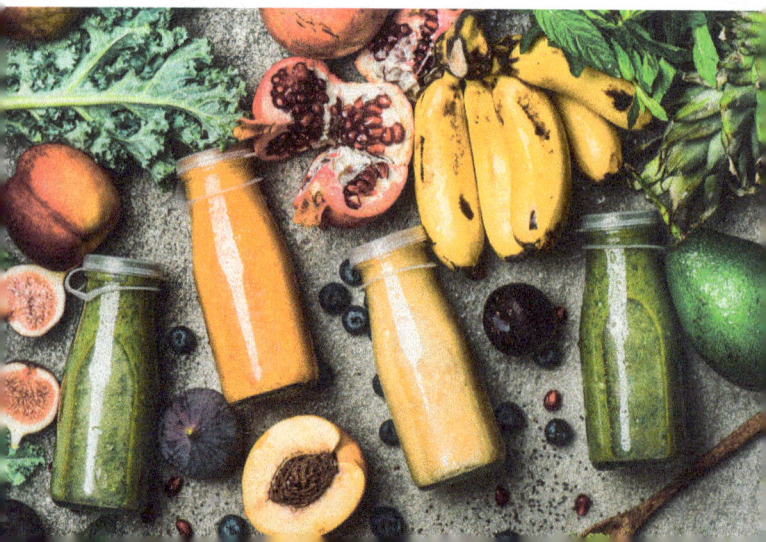

Taking herbs that improve the digestive process (in particular herbs like bitters which are renowned for helping to stimulate the production of bile) is a helpful way to support your liver.

- If the portal vein is overwhelmed and can't deliver clean blood back to the system, cells become malnourished, and waste products such as kidney and gallstones can become a problem.

In this instance, lymphatic or 'blood cleansing' herbs can be used to take some pressure off the liver and help it do its job.

- If the liver can't keep up with the detoxification process, the next largest organ of elimination, the skin, begins to shoulder the burden. Acne, eczema, psoriasis and other skin problems can be compounded because the liver isn't manufacturing or secreting hormones well enough, and valuable nutrients are not being delivered to the cells.

Taking herbs that are known to directly boost liver function can be helpful in the treatment of stubborn skin conditions and menstrual problems.

As the liver has such a wide reaching effect on so many body systems, you can clearly see that improving your liver health can ameliorate many other seemingly unrelated health issues whose cause may be difficult to define.

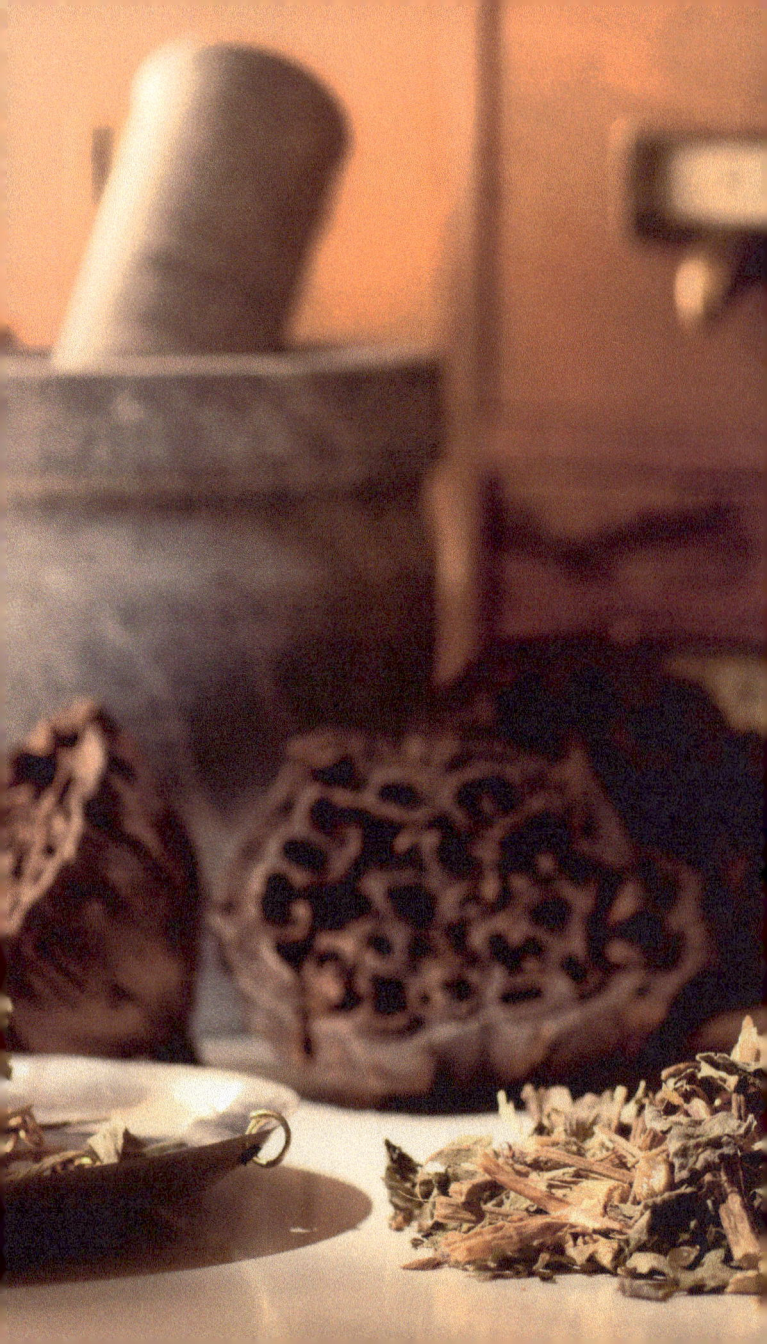

The liver and traditional Chinese medicine

As well as the many physical tasks this amazing organ performs, traditional Chinese practitioners believe that your liver is also responsible for a number of important 'energetic' functions. This idea goes beyond the obvious physical signs and symptoms to describe other subtle influences which affect a person as a whole. In short, good liver health is vital for your emotional wellbeing as well as your physical health.

Liver qi stagnation

Think of your liver as a sort of "army general" whose main job is to regulate the flow of qi (life force) and blood throughout your body. Its main concern is to ensure these energies flow smoothly, evenly and without hindrance.

The liver is very sensitive to anything that disrupts this movement. For example, an excess of negative emotions such as anger can cause the qi to rise, or a traumatic emotional shock can cause the qi to scatter. When qi does not flow smoothly and in the correct way, it can lead to physical problems which can impair the function of the liver. In a practical western sense, this simply means that the liver pathways can become blocked. For example, anger can upset digestive function and shock can delay or even stop menstruation.

Viewed from this perspective, certain emotions are known to 'injure liver qi' impairing function, blocking pathways, and eventually leading to a build-up of toxicity in the system. If these emotions are not properly addressed, you'll soon find yourself paving the way for ill health.

Liver qi stagnation is when the energy of the liver system does not flow as easily and freely as it should. When this happens, different symptoms can occur.

- Pain along the ribs
- Fullness in the upper abdomen
- Irritability
- Moodiness
- Depression
- Anger
- PMS
- Muscular pain
- Stomach ache
- Brittle nails
- Breast distention or tenderness
- Irregular periods
- Sighing
- Bitter taste in mouth
- Feeling of a lump in the throat

In Traditional Chinese Medicine (TCM) this concept is known as 'liver qi stagnation'. As we've already seen, it's a common picture in today's modern society, and expresses itself in the following symptoms:

- Feelings of anger, resentment, moodiness or depression
- PMT
- Nightmares or recurring bad dreams
- Feeling nauseous before 11 am
- 'Floaters' in the line of vision
- Sensitivity to light
- Frequent sighing

Once again we see that improving your liver health can have far reaching effects, not just on the physical body, but also on your mental and emotional wellbeing.

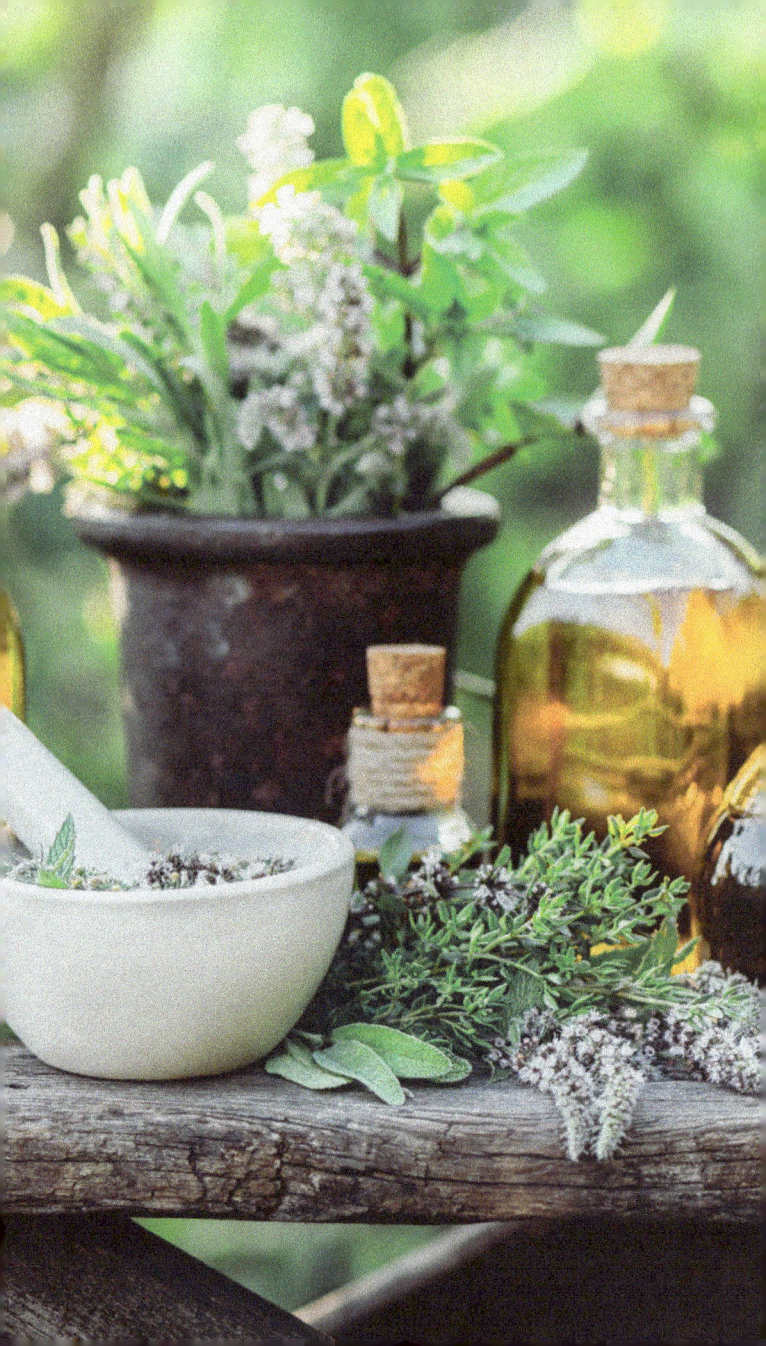

Herbs for liver health

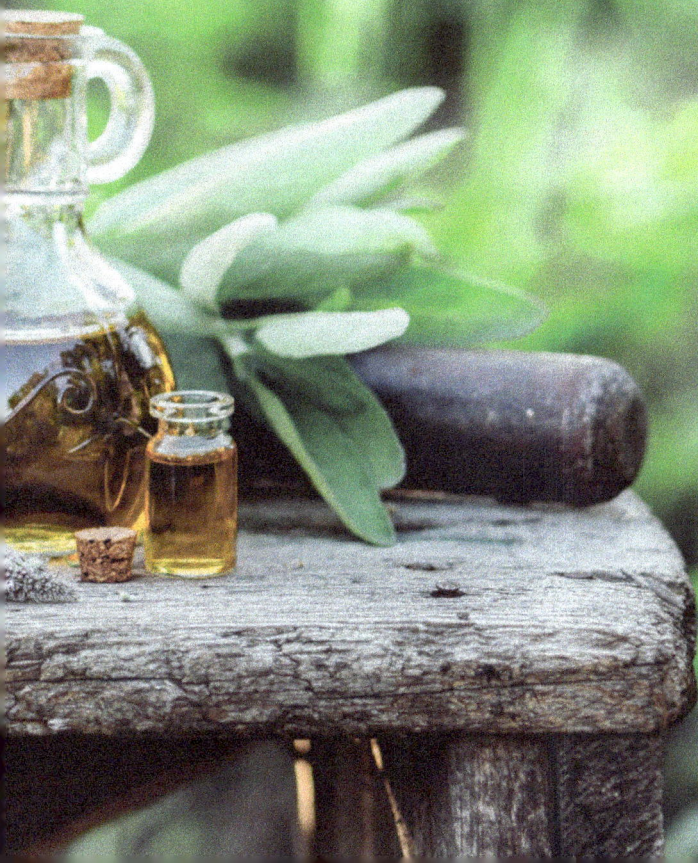

On a practical level, there's a lot you can do to help your liver remain in good form. There are a number of herbs and foods that are very helpful for supporting liver health, both on a physical, and emotional level.

Below is a list of the most frequently used plants in a modern herbal dispensary, most of which are available over the counter and can be taken safely without medical supervision. The majority of these medicines can be purchased from your local herb store or a reputable supplier (a list of recommended companies can be found in the reference section at the end of this book.) It goes without saying that this is far from an exhaustive list, but merely a 'starting point' aimed at signposting you to remedies you might consider to be useful. If you're just beginning on your herbal journey you can regard this list as a 'first port of call'. For more experienced practitioners, it can be viewed as a handy reference tool for recommending herbs to friends and family, or formulating a patient prescription.

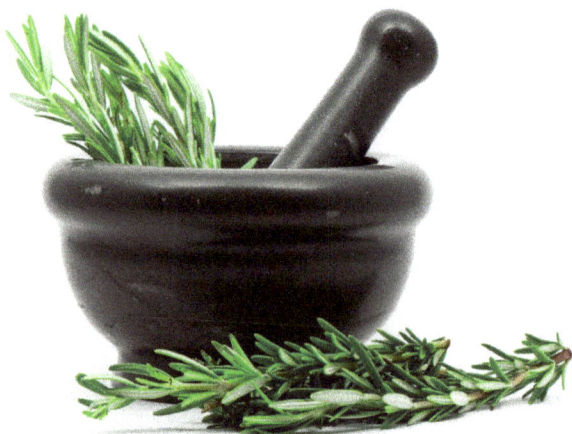

When deciding on which herbs are going to best for your own, or your patient's health, it goes without saying that it is absolutely paramount to take into consideration the individual who is receiving the treatment over and above the condition itself. In this regard, herbal energetics is a crucial consideration. Put simply, if you're providing support to a person who has a hot inflammatory condition, then prescribing hot, dry herbs is likely to aggravate, rather than ameliorate their symptoms.

The subject of herbal energetics is vast, and not within the scope of this book. That being said, it would be remiss not to list the main energetic considerations for each of the plants described, in order that this book serve as a practical and handy starting point from which to explore the most suitable preparations for each individual case. Most good herbal books and monographs will discuss the energetics of each plant remedy. Resources which explore this topic in more detail can be found in the reference section.

If you're unsure if a particular remedy is going to be suitable for you, I recommend paying a visit to your local herbal practitioner. This advice is also extended to practitioners themselves. It can be difficult to be objective when trying to treat oneself, and an alternative viewpoint around treatment plans can be a great learning experience regardless of your level of experience.

On a final note, herbs that are known to be useful in supporting liver health are often referred to under the general title of *hepatics*.

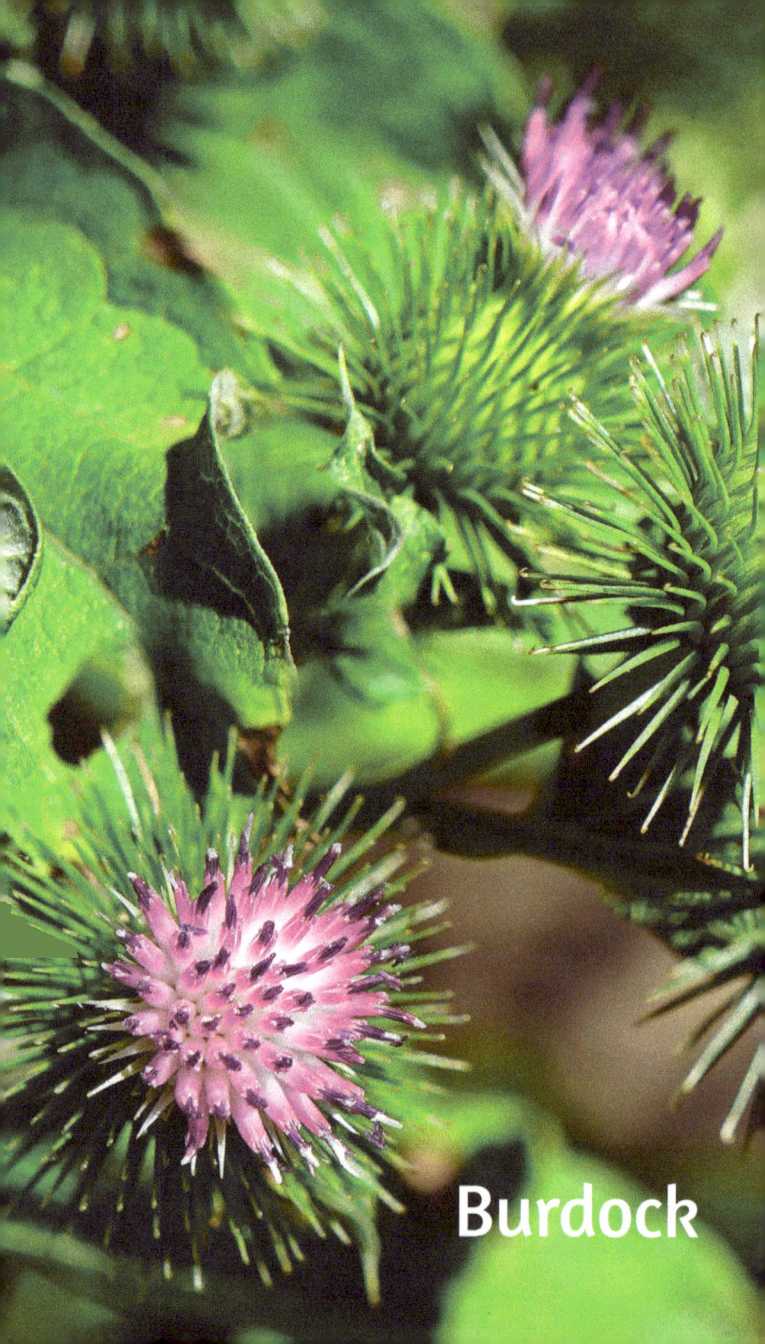

Burdock

Burdock
Arcticum lappa

Energetics
Owing to its nutritive properties, burdock is slightly sweet and nutty with a mildly bitter flavour. It is moistening; slightly oily and pungent, making it suitable for dry, cold conditions.

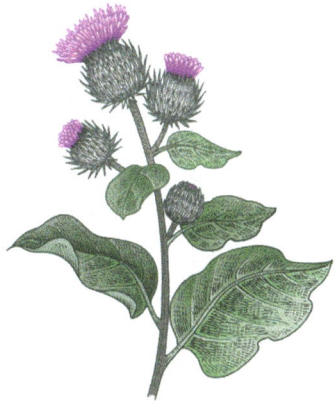

Burdock is useful in deficiency and where there is weakness due to a lack of digestive power. In TCM this is referred to as spleen qi deficiency. The seeds (as opposed to the root) have a demulcent or moistening action, having an affinity for the waters of the body, dispersing them and opening up the channels of elimination. The bitterness of the seeds, roots and leaves increase digestive secretions and have an especially strong impact on the liver. A reliable depurative (it has a powerful purifying action) it relieves wind and stagnation caused by poor digestion.

Burdock combines well with dandelion, providing starches which are necessary for maintaining a healthy gut microbiome. The root is useful in cases of bacterial and fungal infections as it contains fructooligosaccharides which have a probiotic effect.

Burdock also works well with some of the stronger bitter flavours such as gentian, softening and taking

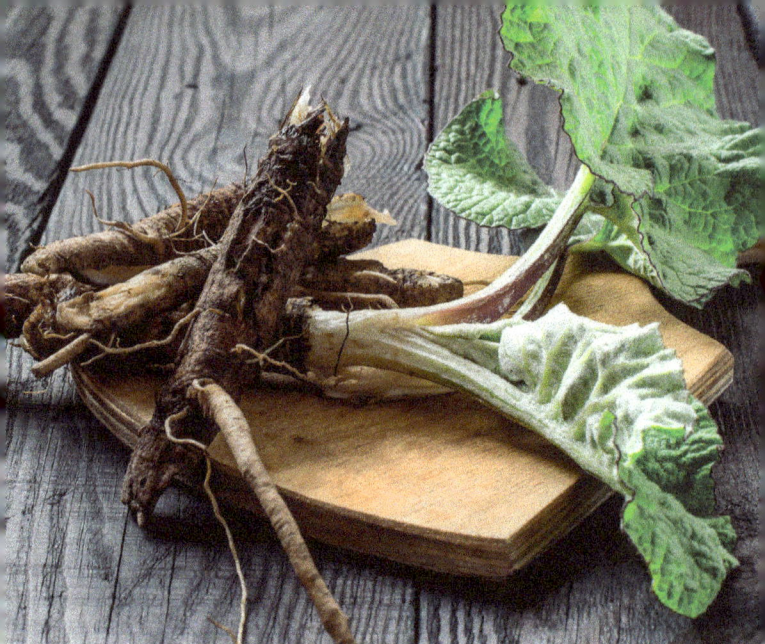

the edge off what can sometimes be too strong a flavour for sensitive types. The root can be chopped and added to soups and stews to create a nutritious bitter stock base (see recipe on page 85).

Burdock is renowned for its blood purifying properties. It improves the action of the sebaceous glands and aids the liver in breaking down hormones. For both these reasons, it is a very useful remedy for acne.

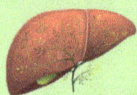

Contraindications
Avoid with anti-diabetic drugs as it can have a hypoglycaemic effect. Use in smaller doses with reactive types.

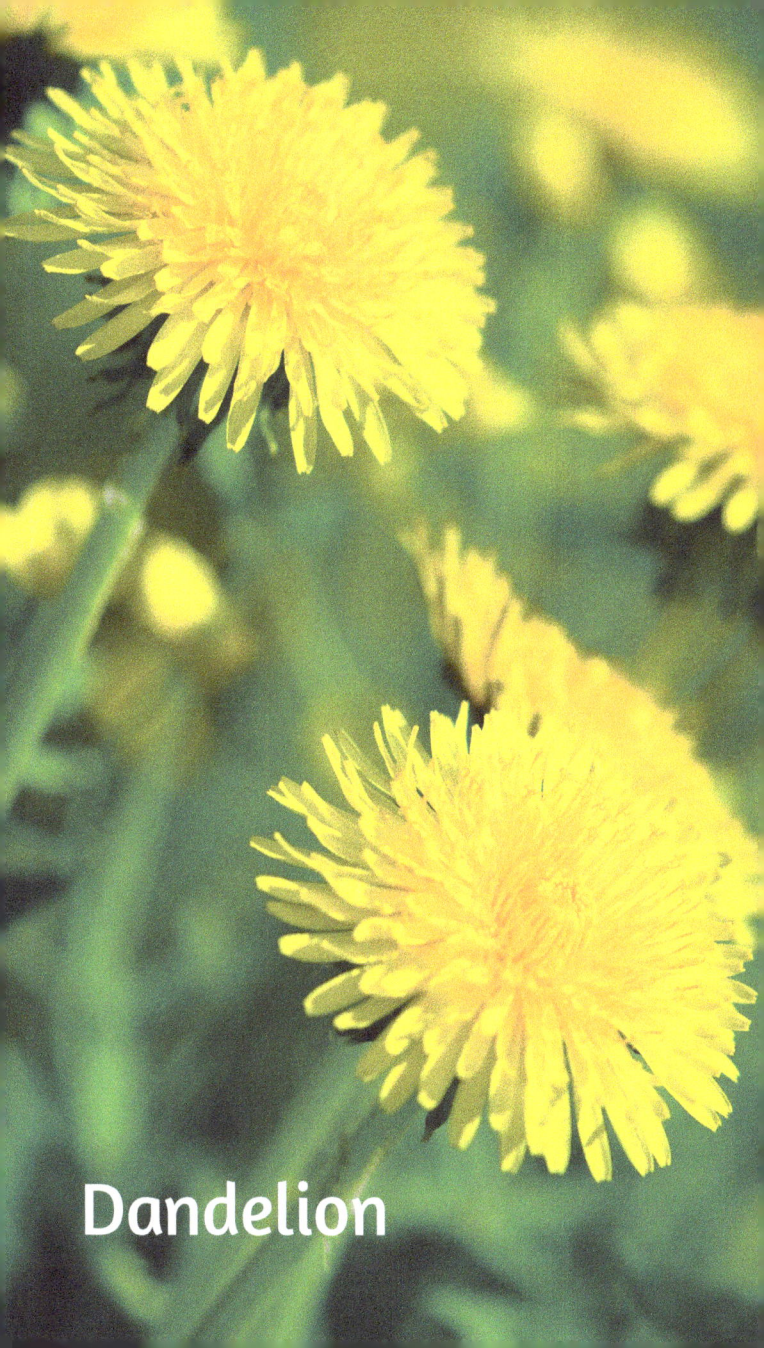

Dandelion

Dandelion
Taraxacum officinale

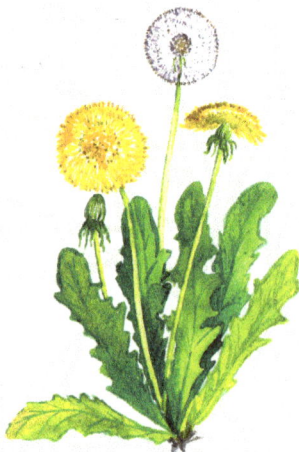

Manufacturers of weed killer products have made millions trying to eradicate this useful plant. Still it comes back, even breaking through concrete to ensure we're able to access its powerful medicine. Dandelion is a useful ally that can be found growing in abundance in most parts of the world. As such, I would encourage you to try this remedy before experimenting with rarer plants that may be threatened by overharvesting. Although it can be exciting to learn about exotic herbs, sometimes the very best remedies can be found in the plants that grow and thrive on your own doorstep.

Dandelion has a wonderful effect on the entire digestive system. It is a very useful plant in the treatment of liver and gallbladder problems, helping to relieve irritability, headaches and nausea related to indigestion. It is a very useful herb in the treatment of constipation, but it does need to be administered in larger more frequent doses. As a gastric tonic, it is valuable in dyspepsia and in cases where there is irritation of the gastric or intestinal membrane.

Dandelion supports the work of both the liver and kidneys in cleansing the bloodstream of impurities. In turn this has an indirect, but beneficial impact on the skin. Dandelion is safe to drink as a tea and makes a useful remedy for clearing skin problems related to hormone imbalances and poor diet. As a food, the young leaves can be added to salad garnishes, the purpose of which has always been to increase digestive juices and help break down the meal on your plate. The bitter leaves help clear the body of waste products which can accumulate in the digestive system.

In France, dandelion is referred to as 'pis-en-lit' (wet the bed) as its diuretic properties are well known. This makes it a useful herb for draining damp and cooling excess heat. It is a beneficial medicine for lymph-oedema and water retention caused by high blood pressure. As it is particularly rich in potassium, it will not deplete valuable minerals in the way that many over the counter medications can.

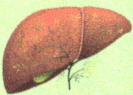

Contraindications
Dandelion should not be used in cases where there is obstruction of the bile duct. Milky latex secretions from the stalk and leaves can cause contact dermatitis. Dandelion extract used in skin creams can help to fade liver spots, but can cause photosensitivity when applied topically.

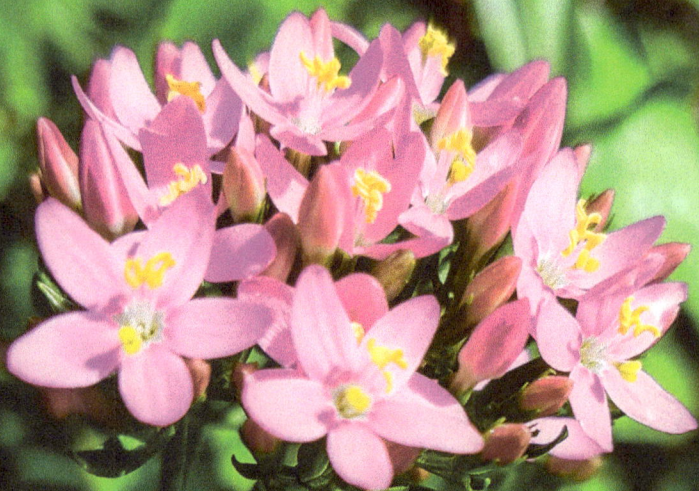

Centaury

Centaury
Centaurium erythraea

Energetics
Aromatic bitter tonic.
Slightly astringent.

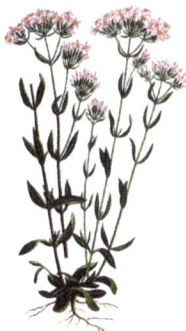

The name of this common weed means 'one hundred pieces of gold' perhaps a reference to its value in treating a wide range of common ailments.

Centaury is traditionally used in the treatment of gastro-intestinal complaints such as bloating, dyspepsia, flatulence, and anorexia. I commonly use this herb in my own practice in cases of heartburn, the cause of which is a lack of tone in the upper sphincter. This causes stomach acid to flow back into the windpipe, usually when the person bends down or is lying in bed at night. Centaury has an astringent, tonifying action, which can make it quite drying. For this reason it combines well with marshmallow root, meadowsweet and chamomile for sour stomach conditions with nausea, vomiting and indigestion. It is especially indicated for appetite loss due to anorexia associated with liver weakness. It is recommended by the 'German Commission E' for people with poor appetite, especially if convalescing after a long illness. Centaury is a good substitute for gentian (the king of bitters) which can be too much of an acquired taste for some people to tolerate. It makes a good base for any bitters formula.

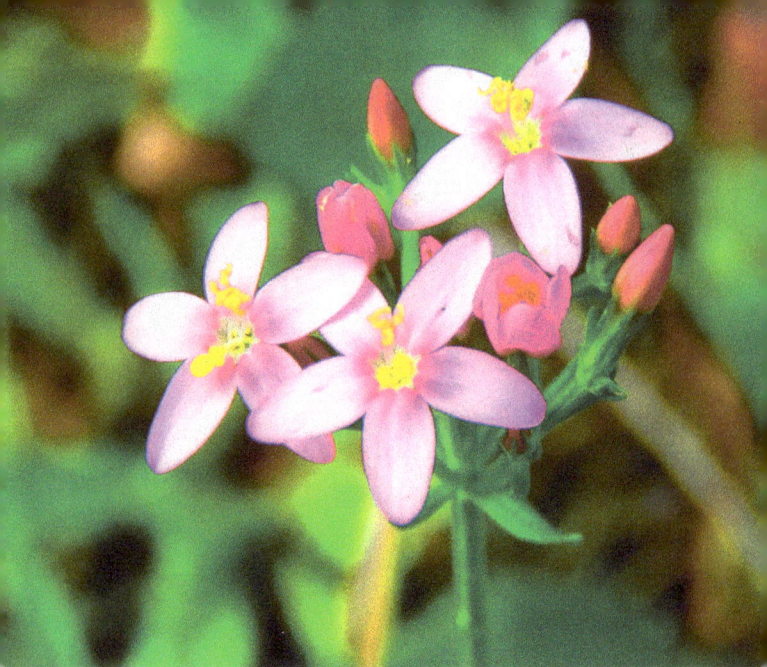

Applied as a lotion, it helps to fade liver spots and chloasma caused by sluggish liver. It is also helpful in cases of tapeworm and kidney stones. In Russia, it is steeped in vodka and drunk as a tonic for liver and gallbladder complaints. It is a common ingredient in many traditional digestive bitter remedies and herbal liqueurs.

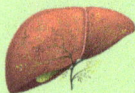

Contraindications
Avoid with peptic ulcers. Not recommended for pregnant or breastfeeding women. In larger doses, it may cause mild abdominal discomfort and cramps.

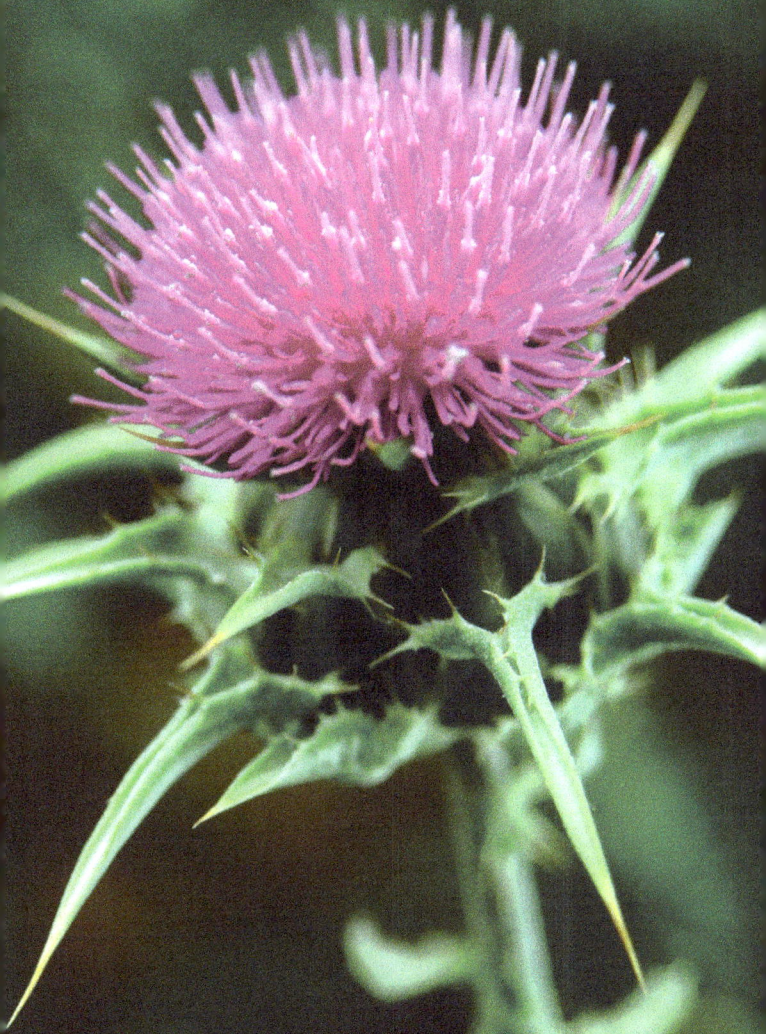
Milk Thistle

Milk thistle
Silybum marianum

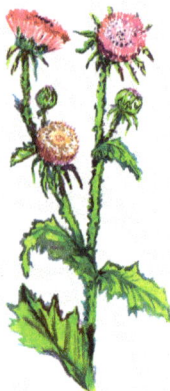

Milk thistle (also known as St. Mary's thistle) is considered to be the 'queen' of all the detoxifying herbs. When it comes to liver health, it is the first plant that most people think of. This is because milk thistle is one of the most studied medicines in the entire herbal materia medica, and has a wealth of scientific data to back up the claims associated with its use.

In studies, milk thistle has been shown to help reduce the build-up of heavy metals, prescription medications, environmental pollutants and alcohol in the liver. It has been used since antiquity for all manner of digestive and liver complaints. In modern times it is employed by herbalists to treat a wide range of chronic and acute liver and gallbladder conditions, including hepatitis, jaundice and cirrhosis. Silymarin, the plant's active ingredient, has both anti-inflammatory and antioxidant properties, increasing the resilience of healthy liver cells and stimulating the repair of those damaged by drugs and alcohol. Its action makes it a useful adjunct for patients undergoing chemotherapy or radiation treatment, as it can help to buffer the negative side effects and aid a speedy recovery.

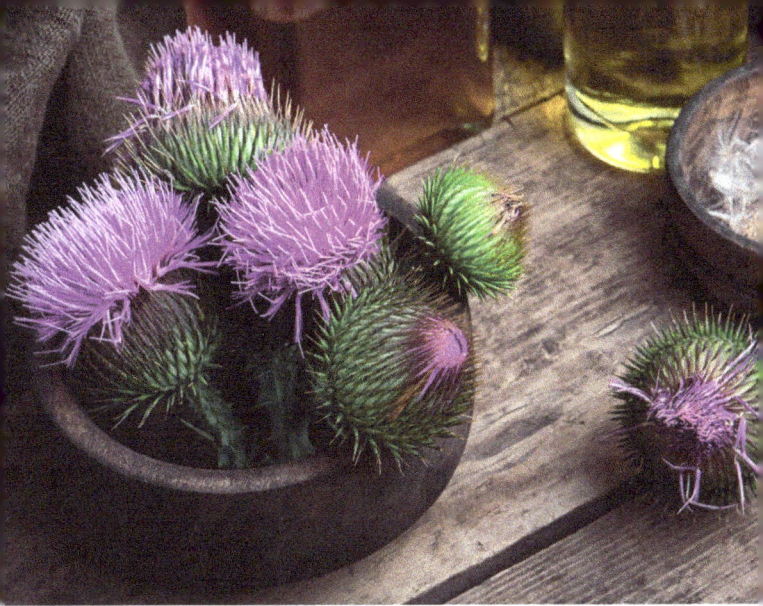

Recent research also indicates that due to its ability to break down fats in the blood, it may be helpful for people who want to lose weight, particularly if the weight gain is associated with type-2 diabetes or insulin resistance. It has strong anti-inflammatory properties which may also make it useful in the treatment of inflammatory skin conditions such as eczema and psoriasis. As these conditions often stem from problems originating in the digestive system, its addition to skin formulations is always worth consideration.

Milk thistle has been documented to prevent fatalities from mushroom poisoning if administered intravenously within 24 hours. The seeds can be eaten freely, and make a nice addition to breakfast cereals or overnight oats.

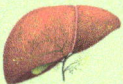

Contraindications
None reported

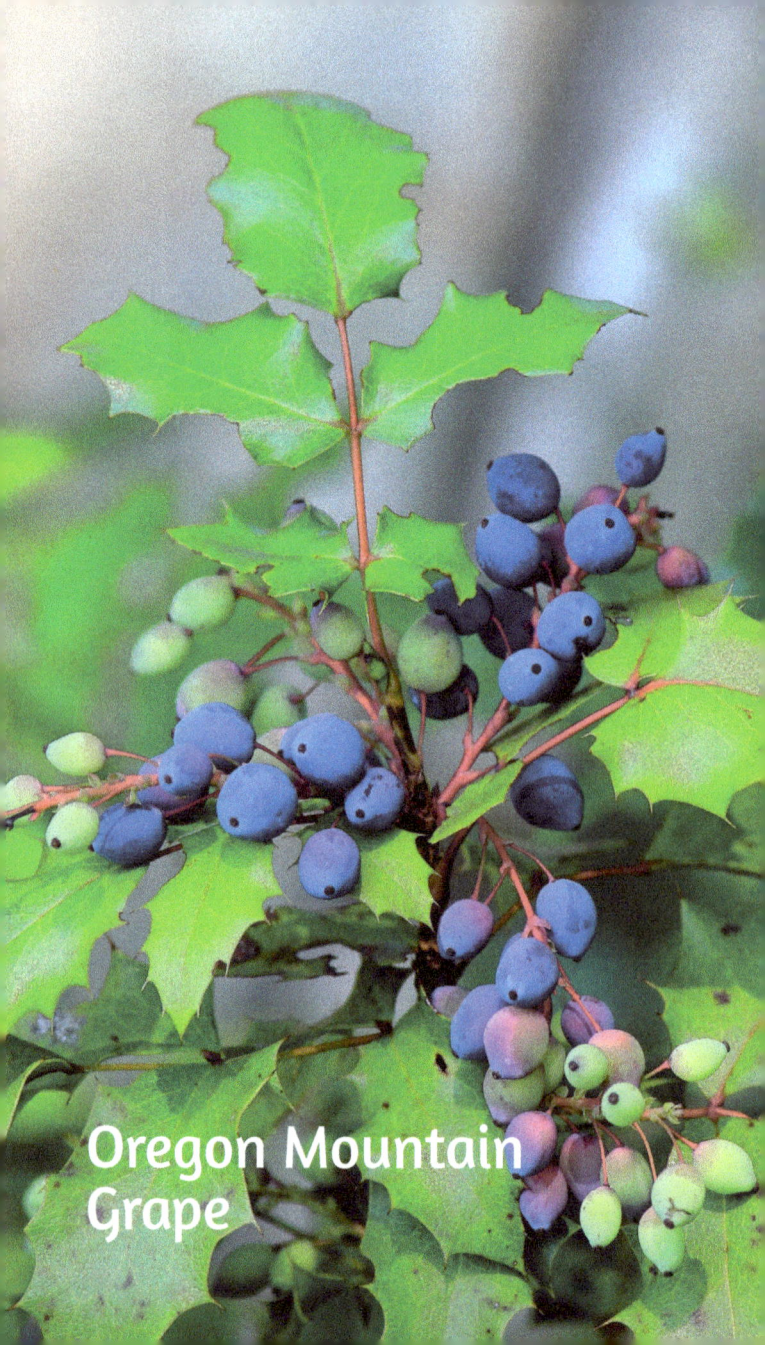

Oregon Mountain Grape

Oregon mountain grape

Berberis aquafolium /
Mahonia aquifolium

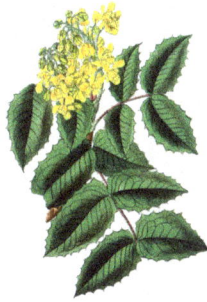

Energetics
Bitter, astringent

Traditionally used by Native American tribes as a detoxifying herb for infections and skin problems, Oregon mountain grape is a bitter herb which has a stimulant action on the secretory glands of the digestive system. It is particularly useful in cases where there is difficulty breaking down and absorbing fats and oils, especially when this leads to constipation.

Used for treating hepatitis and gallstones, Oregon mountain grape has laxative properties. However, unlike plants which contain anthraquinone glycosides* it doesn't directly stimulate peristalsis, but works in a more vitalistic way by acting as a tonic to the whole digestive system. It is useful in cases where there is an accumulation of toxic waste caused by a sluggish metabolism. This may be the root cause of problems which at first glance appear to be unrelated to poor digestive function, such as joint pain, chronic infections, low energy, fatigue, and 'brain fog'.

* Anthraquinone glycosides are phytochemicals that have a potent laxative action. They work by stimulating peristalsis and as such can be irritating to both the upper and lower parts of the gastrointestinal tract. Examples of plants that contain anthraquinone glycosides include aloe vera, senna, cascara sagrada and rhubarb.

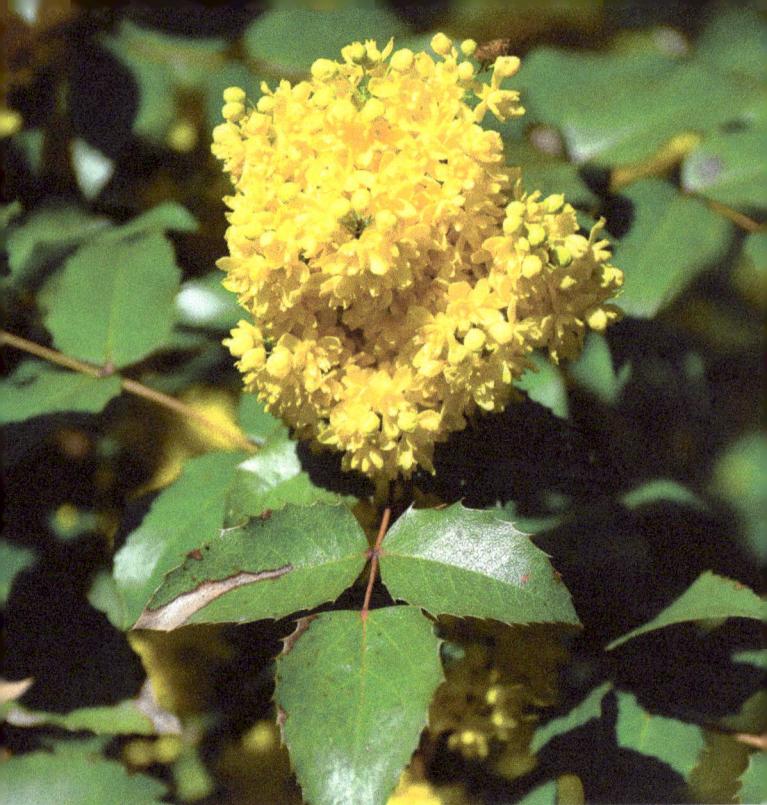

One of the most important applications of Oregon mountain grape root is for chronic skin conditions such as eczema, acne and psoriasis. It helps release stored iron from the liver, making it a useful remedy in cases of anaemia.

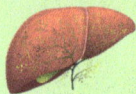

Contraindications
Oregon mountain grape is contra-indicated in hyperthyroidism and during pregnancy.

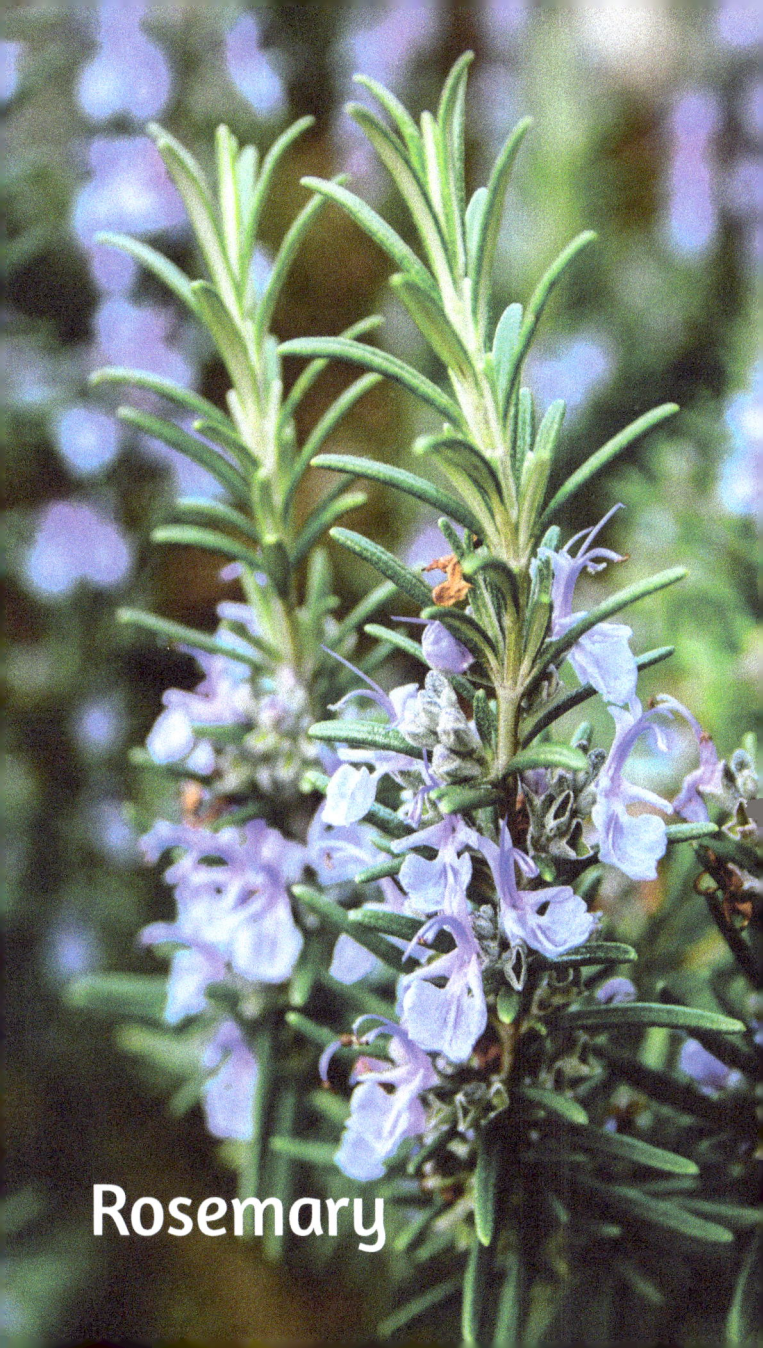

Rosemary

Rosemary

Salvia rosmarinus

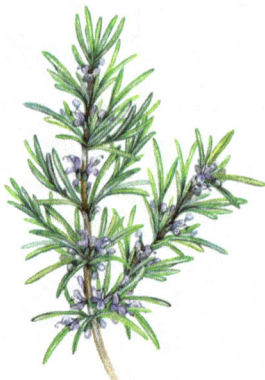

Found in kitchens all over the western world, it's easy to overlook the importance of this valuable plant. Rosemary can be viewed as a 'polycrest' remedy, meaning that it has a very wide range of applications. In fact it's so versatile; it should be a staple in every herbal dispensary.

Rosemary is well known for its reputation as a brain-enhancing memory tonic, but few people realise it also has an amazing capacity for helping the liver remove toxins from the system. A popular culinary herb, it has the ability to stimulate digestion and improve the absorption of nutrients. This action is attributed to its bitter components which help to stimulate bile flow, and the warming volatile oils which stimulate the liver and gallbladder into a greater level of activity. It brings fresh oxygenated blood into the GI tract, helping to warm up and stimulate an underactive, sluggish digestive system.

Rosemary is also used by TCM practitioners as a liver qi relaxant when there is excess tension. It has an interesting biochemical effect, in that it has

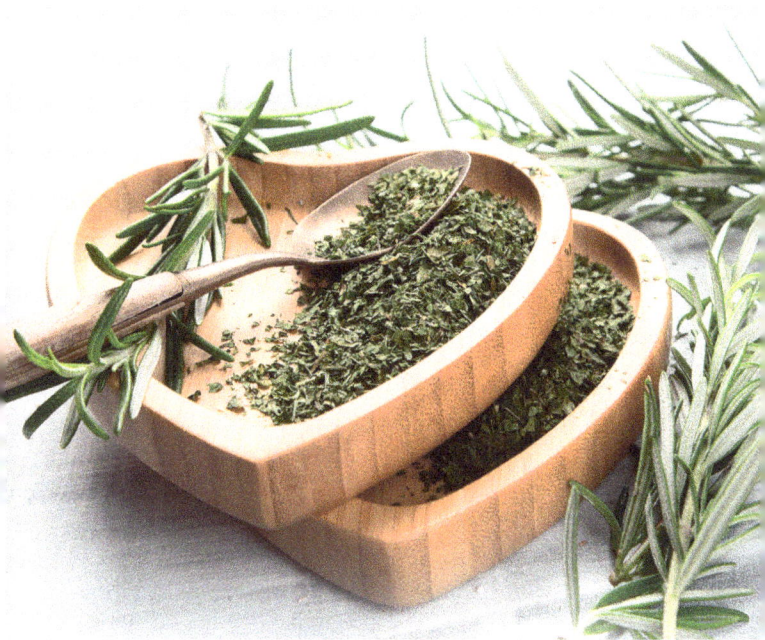

been shown to help the body metabolise cortisol more rapidly.

Rosemary is a fast acting herb, but unlike some of the other, more bitter plants, it has a warm, aromatic flavour and is a pleasant remedy to take. It's a hardy shrub which grows easily in the garden where it needs full sun and well-drained soil. It grows wild in coastal areas (hence its name of Rose-marinus) but thrives best when planted next to its culinary companion Sage (Salvia officinalis).

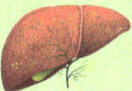

Contraindications
Due to its moving, stimulating properties, Rosemary should be avoided in pregnancy.

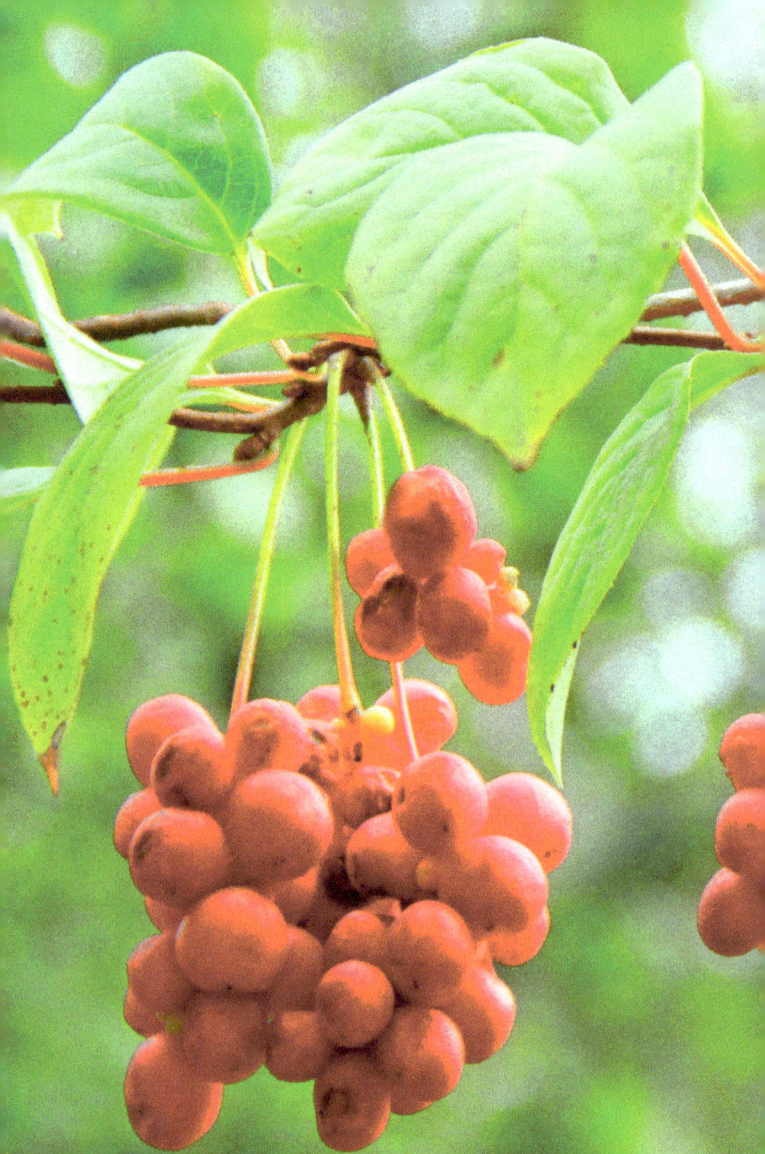

Schisandra

Schisandra

Schisandra chinensis

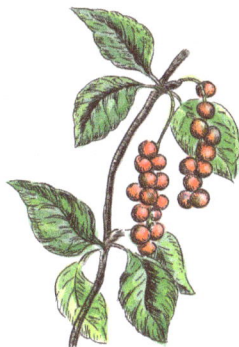

Schisandra is often referred to as the 'five flavoured berry' for the obvious reason that it has the unique trait of having every taste. In Traditional Chinese medicine, the five flavours directly relate to its ability to target the five yin organs of liver, lungs, heart, kidneys and spleen. In western terms, this implies the remedy has the ability to work on all the body's energy centres and influence many systems simultaneously.

Taoist masters call Schisandra the "quintessence of tonic herbs" because it is the only herb in the materia medica that has the following properties:

- Contains all three Treasures (Jing, Qi and Shen)
- Nurtures all five Elements
  (Wood, Fire, Earth, Metal and Water)
- Enters all twelve energy channels (meridians)
  of the human body
- Circulates in the 'extraordinary channels'
- Facilitates the three main 'dan tian'
  (energy centres of the body)
- Is perfectly Yin-Yang balanced

Schisandra is a protective herb, working directly to protect, regenerate and detoxify the liver. The berries have a potent, fast-acting effect, and can metabolise drugs through the system very rapidly. For this reason, it's best avoided by people taking GP prescribed medications for serious health conditions, as it may cause the medicine to be flushed through the system too rapidly.

Like other bitter herbs, the initial taste of the berry stimulates the secretion of digestive enzymes, and the sour flavour helps to increase saliva, which is necessary for emulsifying carbohydrates and fats.

Modern research has shown that Schisandra berries act as adaptogens (herbs which help to increase stamina and endurance under times of stress.) For this reason, the remedy is a boon for anyone whose liver and digestive functions are impaired due to stress.
Schisandra works well as a high strength tincture or fluid extract, either on its own or combined with other vitamin C rich herbs such as hibiscus or roses. It also combines well with mushrooms such as reishi, lion's mane and turkey tail, amplifying their medicinal effect. This combination works very well for people who are convalescing after radiation therapy (which has a very damaging effect on the liver.)

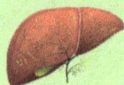

Contraindications
Avoid in pregnancy and epilepsy

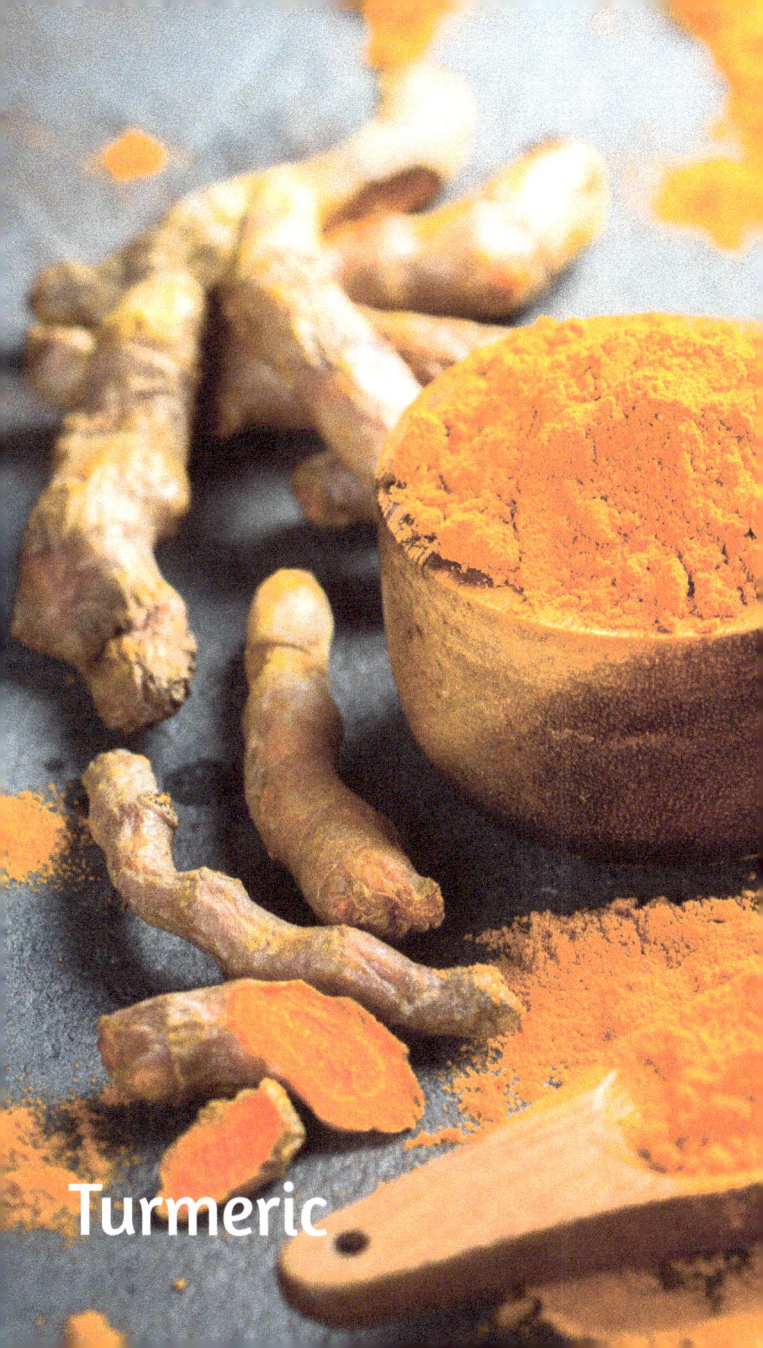

Turmeric

Turmeric

Curcuma longa

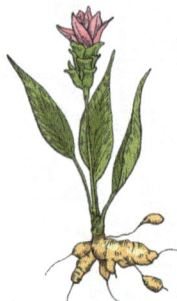

The cousin of ginger, turmeric has long been held in high esteem for its many varied medicinal properties. It is well known for its antioxidant properties, and for its incredible ability to help modulate the inflammatory response. However few people realise that turmeric is also an excellent chologue with an impressive ability to support liver health.

When taken with a meal, the spice triggers bile flow (which as we have seen, is necessary for digesting fats). It achieves this by stimulating the muscles of the gallbladder and increasing the output of digestive enzymes produced by the pancreas.

Turmeric generates the secretion of specialist enzymes which assist the liver in breaking down and metabolising toxic substances. It is also able to release excess iron stored in the liver, and so may be helpful in cases of anaemia.

One teaspoon of powdered turmeric taken twice daily in a small amount of water lessens the symptoms of PMS by activating liver function which in turn helps regulate the hormones. The medicinal effect of turmeric can be enhanced up to 20 times by combining it with ginger and black pepper.

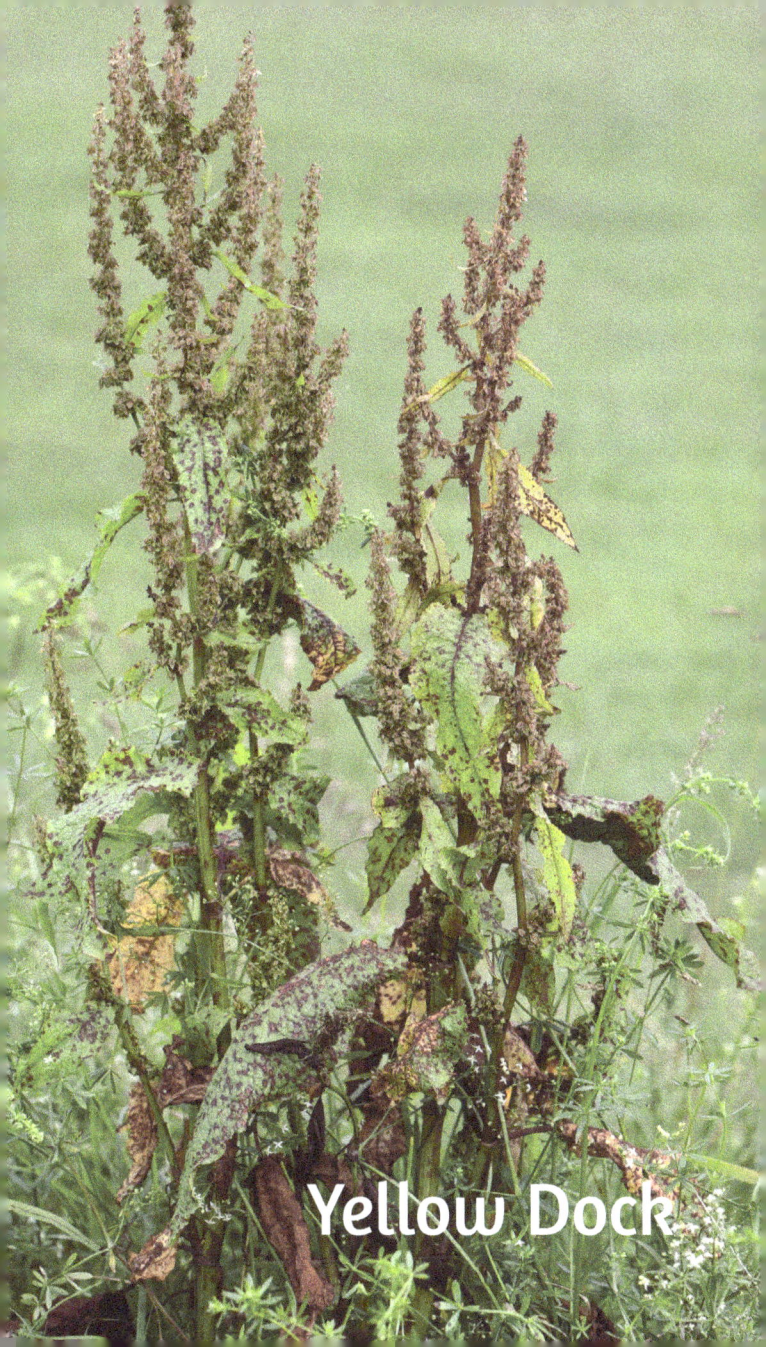

Yellow Dock

Yellow dock

Rumex crispus

Energetics
Cool, bitter.

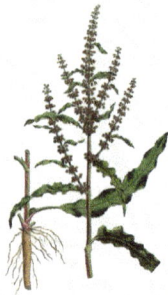

Yellow dock is a common sight among hedgerows and along roadsides in temperate areas. It's a bitter tonic, working in a similar way to Oregon mountain grape root, by stimulating the production of bile and the flow of digestive juices. It does contain some anthraquinone glycosides, but has a milder action than other more purgative, laxative herbs.

The root has the special ability to draw iron from the soil, which is then assimilated by the plant and transmuted into a bio-available and easy to assimilate from. Herbalists have been known to sprinkle iron filings on the soil over land where it grows in order to enhance the blood enriching quality of the plant. The tall spiky flowers have an almost "rusty" appearance, which according to the doctrine of signatures gives a clear indication for its medicinal use.* It is a very useful plant for people suffering from iron deficient anaemia. As it also contains sulphur, it makes an invaluable addition to any formula aimed at supporting people with chronic skin conditions.

*The doctrine of signatures purports that herbs resembling various parts of the body can be used to treat ailments of those corresponding organs. It is a curiosity that many liver remedies have yellow flowers, alluding to the fact that they are helpful in the manufacture of bile.

It is helpful in cases of jaundice, shingles, and painful boils, and combines well with blue flag root and dandelion for dry, itchy skin complaints. It helps to clear heat and is useful for headaches relating to poor digestion. Yellow dock is a traditional pot herb. The leaves are added to stews to make the meat tender and to help the dish cook more quickly.

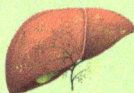

Contraindications
Large doses can cause gastric disturbance and nausea.

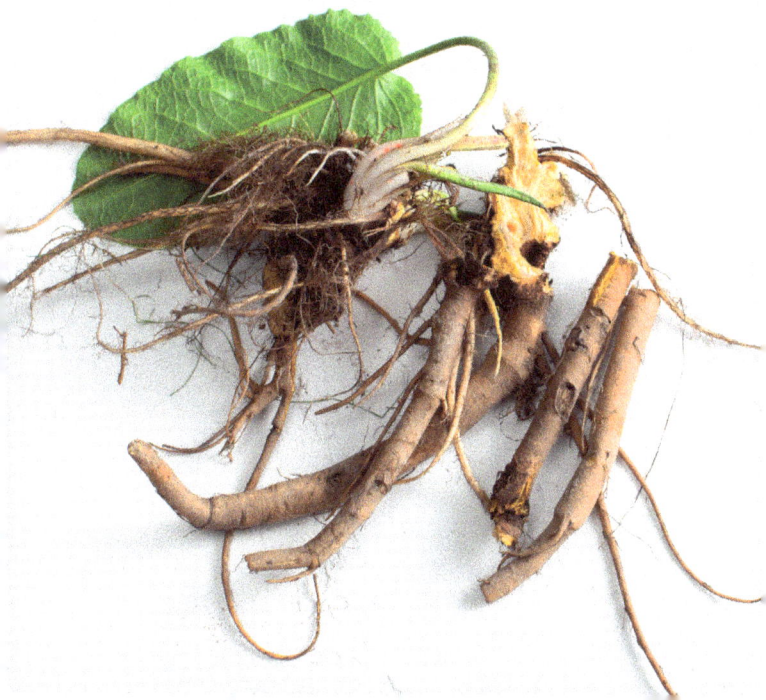

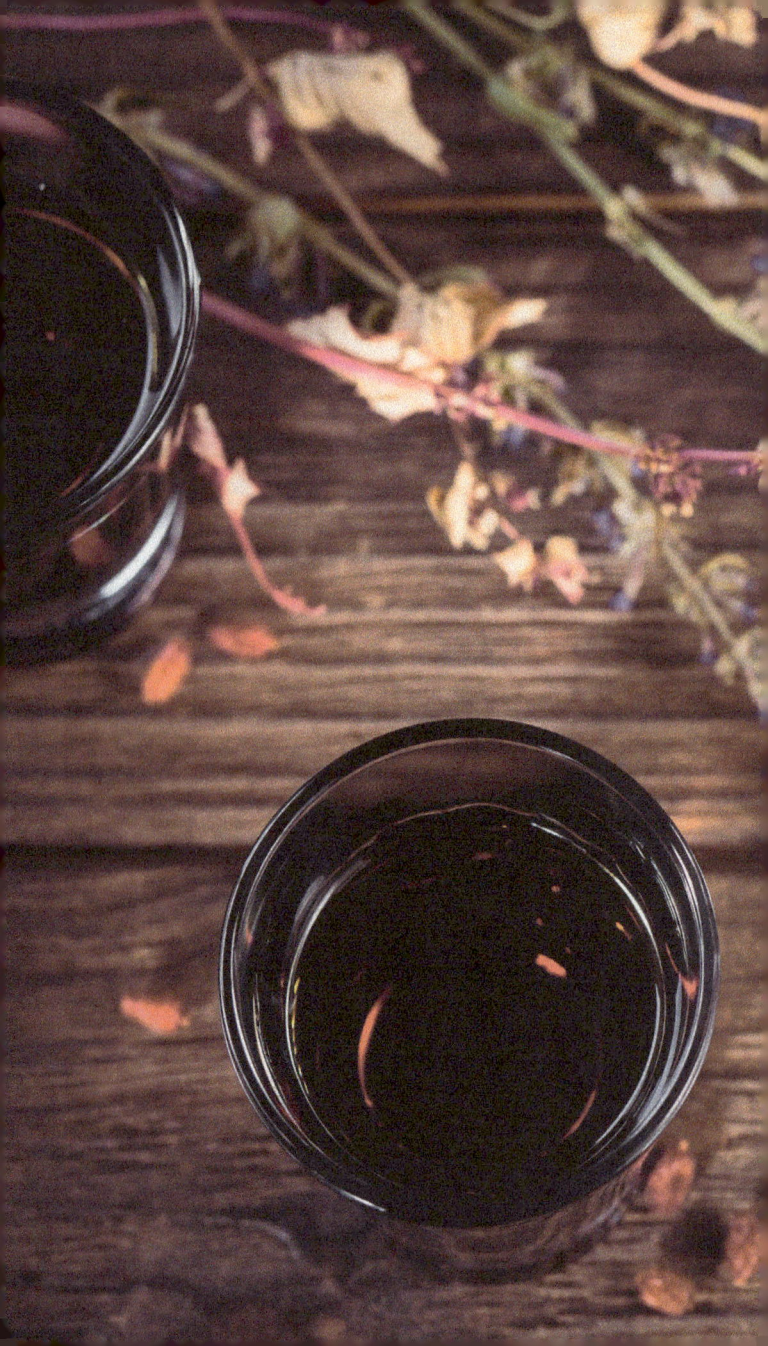

Bitters for liver health

You may have noticed that all the herbs we've discussed so far have one thing in common. They each have what we might loosely describe as a 'bitter flavour profile'. There's a very good reason for this. Bitter taste receptors are found throughout the body and are directly stimulated by bitter flavours; something we don't tend to get a lot of in our modern western diet.

Try this experiment

Close your eyes and imagine you're squeezing the juice of a lemon onto your tongue. Can you feel your saliva glands going to work? This is an example of how bitter flavours signal to your body that food is on the way. The receptors acknowledge the signal and produce the digestive enzymes needed to break down the food being ingested.

Your liver is a fundamental part of your digestive system. As we've already seen, one of its jobs is to produce bile (a sort of 'washing up liquid') which helps your body to break down fats. For centuries people have used what nowadays we might refer to as 'bitter tonics' to help this process along. Essentially, bitter tonics are herbal remedies that 'get your digestive juices flowing'.

You may already be familiar with bitters without even realising it. Here are a few examples you've probably come across.

- Angostura Bitters - traditionally kept behind the bar to settle upset stomachs
- Bitter Melon - often served in India as an accompaniment to food
- Tonic Water - contains quinine, a bitter substance made from the bark of the Cinchona tree

A study carried out at the University of Pavia in Italy showed that participants who took a shot of herbal bitters before eating experienced increased weight loss, reduced their cholesterol, and had lower blood sugar levels than those who didn't. This is because herbal bitters increase the secretion of enzymes which help you to digest your food. Interestingly, they also directly affect the hormones which control your appetite.

Bitter herbs of this nature generally fall into one of two categories:

1. Those that stimulate the production of bile salts (choleretics)	For example Oregon mountain grape and black root (Leptandra virginica.)
2. Those that stimulate the flow of bile from the liver causing the gallbladder to contract (cholagogues)	For example burdock, greater celandine and yellow dock

Both categories of herbs are useful in aiding the proper elimination of toxins.

Herbalists have long used the properties of bitter herbs such as gentian, angelica, wormwood and centaury to create classic digestive formulas and bitter tonics. One of the most famous of these formulas is Swedish bitters.

The recipe for Swedish bitters is reputed to be based on an original formula devised by Paracelsus, a 16th Century alchemist. It was made popular by Maria Treben in her famous book 'Health through God's Pharmacy' which was published in 1980 and reputed to have sold over 6 million copies around the world. The book suggests a wide range of uses for the preparation, from the treatment of acne to helping improve your child's school reports! Although some of the claims are quite entertaining, it is in fact a very reliable and helpful remedy for the relief of symptoms related to poor liver function. It makes a handy digestive tonic for occasions such as Christmas, where there is a tendency to over burden the digestive system with rich food and drink.

Swedish bitters is one of the most requested pre-mix blends stocked in my own dispensary. When purchasing Swedish bitters, always ensure you buy the alcohol extract. Some products are extracted in vegetable glycerine and so have a "sweet" taste, which is counterintuitive to the bitter action required for the herbs to truly be effective.

Information about stockists can be found in the resources section at the end of this book.

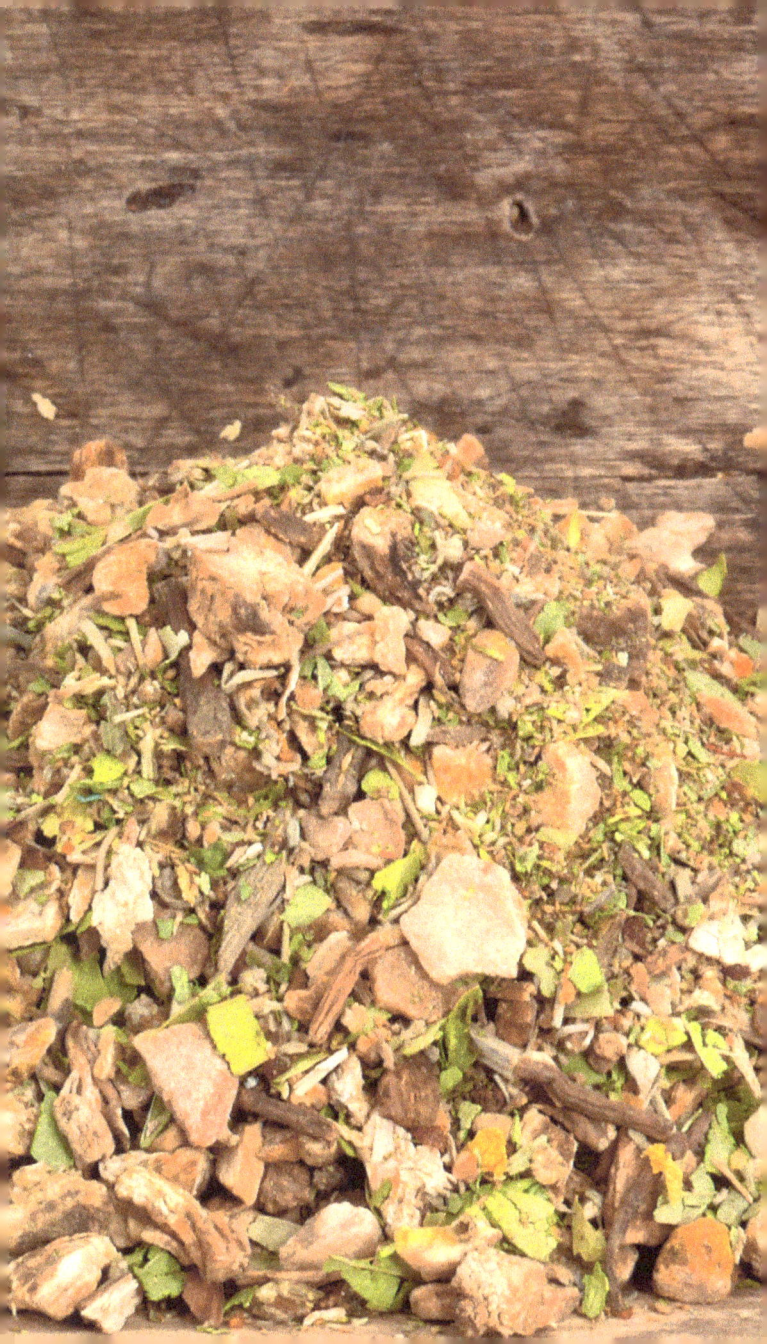

Dark and Stormy Mushroom Bitters

The following is a twist on the classic bitters formula. It relies on the bitter taste of the mushrooms to stimulate the production of digestive enzymes. The original formula was first published by Christopher Hobbs in his informative book 'Medicinal mushrooms: an exploration of tradition, healing and culture' and republished by the Herbal Academy (a link to the original article can be found in the reference section.)

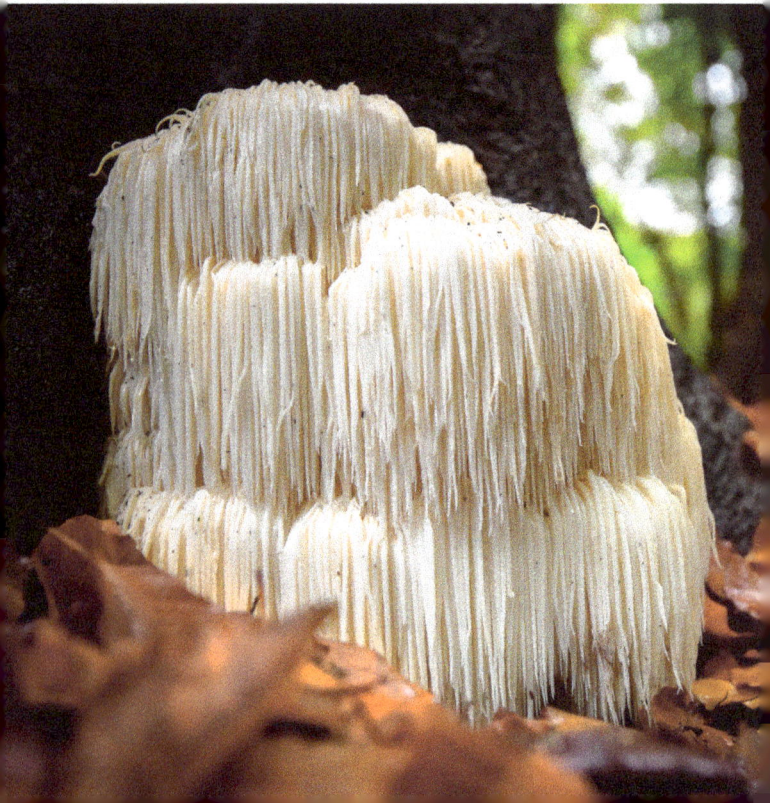

The following formula is my own take on the recipe, and has proved to be very popular with clients at the clinic.

Common name	Latin name	Dose (ml)
Reishi	Ganoderma lucidum	25
Turkey tail	Corioulus versicolor	20
Lion's mane	Hericium erinaceus	15
Damiana	Turnera diffusa	15
Bitter orange glycerite	-	15
Cardamom seed	Elletaria cardamomum	5
Liquorice root	Glycyrrhiza glabra	5
Ginger	Zingiber officinalis	10 drops to taste

Dose

Take 20 drops in a little warm water before meals. Use up to 3 ml 2-3 times daily for additional support. Its orangey taste makes it also a nice addition to sparkling water, cocktails, or mocktails.

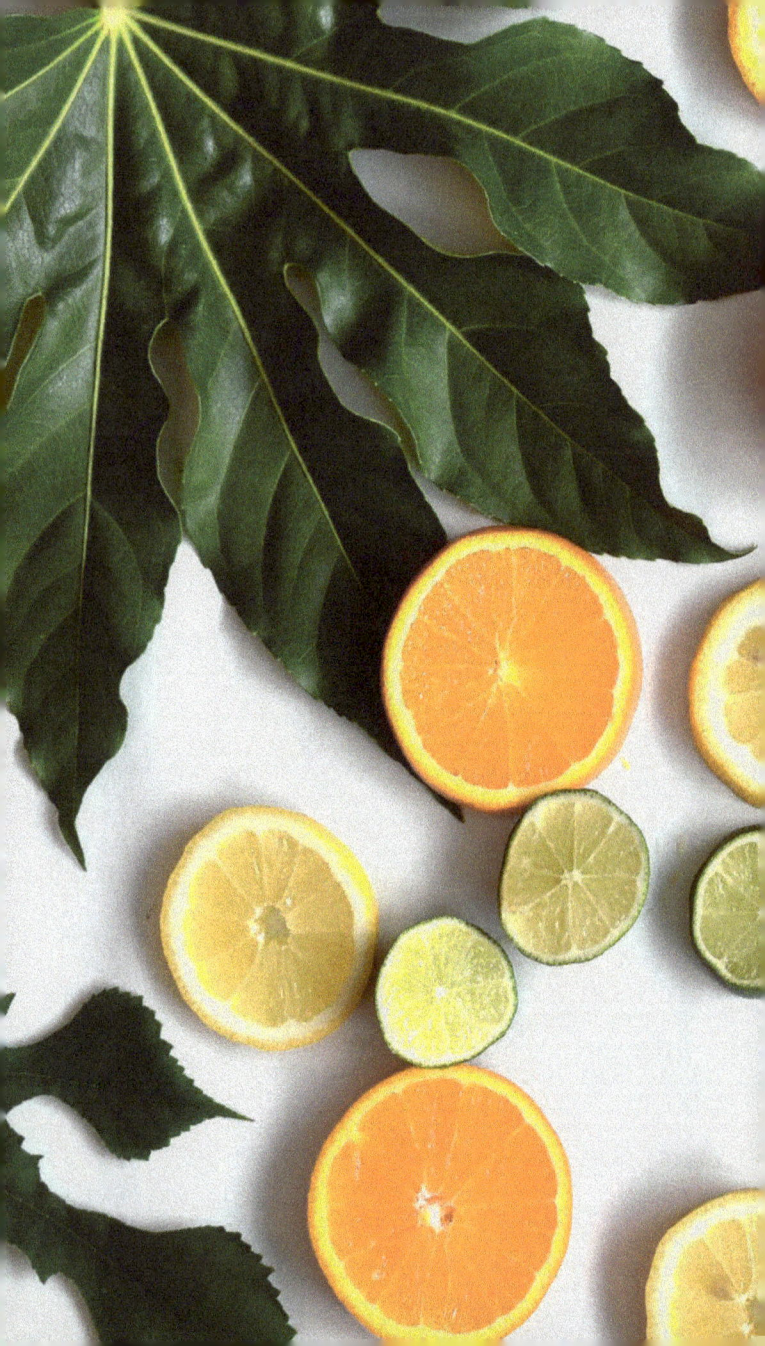

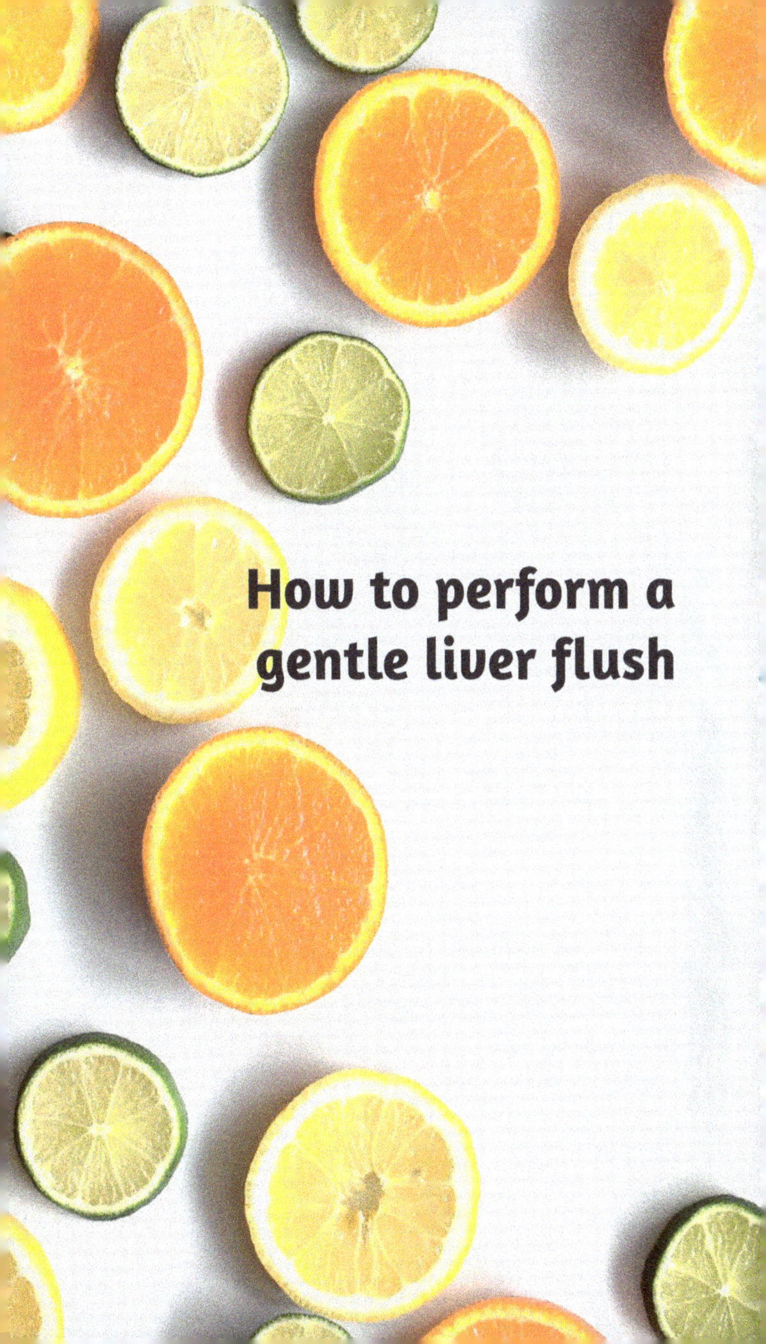

How to perform a gentle liver flush

As well as ensuring you get your daily dose of supportive herbs, the practice of liver flushing is also very beneficial for your general wellbeing.

It's a remarkable fact that almost all of the blood in your body passes through your liver every three to four minutes. In the process of removing toxic by-products from food and environmental pollutants, some of this waste is released into the digestive tract via the bile duct. This is why bitter herbs that stimulate the flow of bile are an essential

Liver flushing achieves the following objectives

- Drains accumulated toxins, cholesterol, and other stagnant waste from the vital organs

- Improves bile flow and motility of the gallbladder

part of the detoxification process. We can use this principle to perform what herbalists and naturopaths refer to as a 'liver flush,' a simple and effective way to improve your liver and digestive health.

Liver flushing is recommended by herbalists the world over. Undertaking a flush gently encourages the liver to improve its excretory function by eliminating old bile that may be trapped inside the ducts, and moving any stagnant material out from the gallbladder.

Performing a short liver flush at the change of season (or whenever you're in need of a boost), is a great way to feel better and rapidly recharge your energy levels.

Why is liver flushing beneficial for health?

Many of the chemicals and toxic compounds found in modern environmental pollutants are fat soluble. This means they can hang around in your body's fat deposits 'in storage' until the time comes when you have a chance to deal with them. For the vast majority of people, unless they make a conscious effort to undertake a program of detoxification, the opportunity to rest and digest rarely comes around.

One of the liver's jobs is to store fat, the source of which is excess sugar circulating in the bloodstream. To maintain homeostasis, this excess blood sugar is converted into glycogen and dumped in the liver where it's kept on hand for emergency stores of energy. This is how a fatty liver develops. Because toxins are stored in fat, the liver itself can begin to get toxic.

Doing a short liver flush from time to time prevents the accumulation of waste deposits in the system, and has a huge range of health benefits including:

- Improved digestion (helpful for people with gallbladder issues who are unable to properly digest fats)
- Reduce cholesterol
- A harmonising effect on the menstrual cycle
- Improved skin conditions
- Relief of constipation caused by a lack of bile and digestive juices
- Increased energy
- The releases of old negative emotions such as anger and resentment

How does it work?

The liver detoxifies chemicals by turning them from fat soluble to water soluble so they can be excreted via the kidneys (urine) or the skin (sweat). During this complicated process, some waste is also released into the digestive tract via the bile duct. We've already seen that herbs which stimulate bile flow promote detoxification. Doing a short liver flush increases the flow of bile, allowing the body to dump the toxins which are stored in the liver into the digestive tract, ready for elimination via the gut.

Is liver flushing safe?

Herbalists and healers have performed cleanses since the year dot. In fact many cultures embrace the idea of cleansing - the concept of giving your body a chance to rest is really nothing new. Native Americans have their sweat lodges, Muslims fast during Ramadan, and here in the West we think nothing of taking a sauna, having a massage, or sweating it out on the sports field. Why would we universally choose to do these things if they didn't make us feel good? The following cleanse is the one I use with my patients here at my own clinic. I've completed it hundreds of times (including on myself). Although there are innumerable ways to perform a liver flush, I like this approach because it's based around a traditional, tried and tested method that's gentle enough to be tolerated by most people who are in a reasonably good state of health.

Before you go ahead and try the methods described, there are one or two important points to note. Carrying out a liver flush may not be suitable for people who have gallstones or serious liver conditions such as cancer or hepatitis. Although some practitioners recommend liver flushing for the removal of gallstones (if you have the stomach for it, check out YouTube to see some truly fascinating photographs and accounts of the process,) due to the possibility of the stones becoming impacted, I personally wouldn't take the gamble without the supervision of an extremely experienced practitioner.

It also goes without saying that a liver flush should never be performed by pregnant or breastfeeding women. It's also important to remember that the effectiveness of any GP prescribed drugs you may be taking can be reduced when performing a flush. This is because your medication will pass through your system much more quickly than usual. All this can have big implications if you're taking medicine for serious conditions.

If you're at all unsure, the general rule is to check with your doctor before carrying out ANY naturopathic cleanse at home. If at all possible, find a practitioner who is experienced in cleansing to work with you and supervise your program. Remember: when it comes to detoxing, one size does not fit all. The length of time needed will vary from person to person. Factors such as your age, your current state of health, and whether or not you've done this kind of thing before, should all be taken into account.

As I said, there are many different variations of the liver flush; however, the following method is gentle enough for the first time cleanser, while still offering deeply healing benefits for more experienced detoxers. Should you be interested in learning more about this topic, further resources can be found in the reference section at the end of the book.

Performing the flush

For peace of mind, the flush should be done in the comfort of your own home on a day when you have no appointments or other responsibilities.

You will need:

- The juice of one whole lemon
- Half a pint (250 ml) of organic apple juice
- 1 tablespoon of cold pressed, extra virgin olive oil
- 1 clove of garlic
- A small piece of fresh ginger root
- A teaspoon of organic turmeric powder

Each ingredient has been chosen for a very specific purpose and so it's very important not to deviate from the recipe by adding or switching out any of the above.

Apple juice

The malic acid contained in apple juice renders toxic metals inert and increases cellular energy. The addition of freshly squeezed organic juice has the added benefit of improving the flavour of the drink.

Olive oil

When the liver encounters oil it reacts by producing bile. The addition of olive oil to the drink will stimulate the body to produce large amounts of bile, which then pass into the small intestine. This is how the flush helps to remove toxic waste.

Lemon

The sour taste activates digestive enzymes. Like apple juice, it helps to improve the flavour of the drink.

Garlic

Although very anti-social, garlic is one of the key ingredients in the flush so please don't be tempted to omit it! Garlic contains sulphur compounds which are crucial for the detoxification process.

Ginger

Ginger contains a compound known as gingerol, a chemical that is known to counteract liver toxicity by stimulating bile excretion. The addition of ginger settles the stomach and helps to prevent nausea.

Turmeric

Turmeric is one of the most anti-inflammatory substances found in nature. Curcumin, the active ingredient found in turmeric, is a very powerful detoxifier.

In addition to the above ingredients, you'll also need some herbal detox tea to drink after you consume the flush. You can make this up yourself using a combination of the following dried herbs:

Fennel, Nettle, Dandelion, Liquorice, Cinnamon and Cardamom.

Alternatively pick up a pre made blend from your local health food shop or supermarket. There are a number of really good brands available which market their products as detox teas — just be sure they only contain dried herbs and are sugar free. My personal favourite is the Yogi Tea label due to the quality and flavour of the herbal blends (and also the price).

Method

Finely chop the garlic and ginger. Use a mincer or fine grater if you have one. The smoother the bits, the easier it will be to get down.

Add all the ingredients to a Nutri Bullet or food mixer and pulse until you have a smooth, thick liquid. Consume the drink immediately, followed by two cups of lukewarm herbal detox tea which you will have prepared in advance.

The liver flush should be performed first thing in the morning on an empty stomach. It's important to leave at least one hour before eating in order to allow the flush to work its way through your digestive tract unimpeded.

What to expect

The effects of the liver flush will be different for everyone, and is entirely dependent on the health of your liver, digestive system and your own individual physical and emotional makeup. I've performed the process innumerable times, and each time I've experienced a different outcome. The following is a general guide of what to expect if this is your first ever flush.

Feelings of tiredness are quite common. This is because your liver is working hard to move toxins through the system and requires extra energy to perform this job. The fact that toxicity and stagnant waste material is being mobilised back into the system ready for elimination can also make you feel sluggish. Any tiredness should quickly pass, and most people report feeling increased energy and vitality very soon after they finish the flush. To avoid any unnecessary stress, always ensure you undertake the cleanse on a day where you're able to take time to rest and digest.

During a cleanse avoid:

- Sugar and highly processed foods
- Refined oils which are heating to the liver
- Chemicals in household and personal care products
- Stress
- Alcohol

People who have a high level of congestion may also feel slightly nauseous. Drinking ginger tea can help to reduce any queasiness. Due to the fact that bile is being moved rapidly through the system, it is also common to experience loose stools. You may feel the need to pass an urgent bowel motion (although this doesn't happen to everyone).

Bile and toxins aren't the only things that move when cleansing the liver. Many people also experience a shift of emotions. You may feel extra sensitive, or have feelings of anger or upset during, or shortly after the cleanse. In the past I've had clients who reported feeling more intuitive or who had vivid dreams. This is an example of stagnant emotions being released from the system and is quite normal. Although most people find this a welcome release, if you have a lot of issues going on in your life it may be an uncomfortable process. If you're at all worried about the emotional aspect of the flush, it may be prudent to wait for a time where things are more settled before undertaking the cleanse. Alternatively enlisting emotional support in the form of friends, family, or even a counsellor may be helpful so you can feel fully supported throughout the process. Releasing stuck emotions can be unpleasant, but can also be very beneficial, especially if these emotions are injuring your liver qi and causing physical symptoms.

For all of the above reasons, it's important to consider the timing, the environment, and your energy levels before deciding to undertake a liver flush. Be prepared, get support and do your homework so you can gain the most benefit from your experience.

How often should you flush?

How long is a piece of string? For some people one flush is enough to regain their energy and feel brighter, other people may feel a need to go deeper, or have long standing health concerns which would benefit from a longer cleanse.

If this is your first time doing a liver flush, I suggest trialling it out for one day in order to gauge your reaction. Give yourself a break for a few days, and if you feel the need to repeat the cleanse you can then go ahead and undertake a short program.

My personal recommendation would be to flush for a period of between seven to ten days. I have found this to be the optimal time frame. Any longer and you risk changing your bowel habits, depleting your energy, or upsetting the delicate balance of your gut microbiome. That said, I know practitioners who recommend performing the flush in 10 day cycles (10 days on, and 3 days off as needed). Listen to your body and do what feels right for you. As with all things in life, moderation is the key.

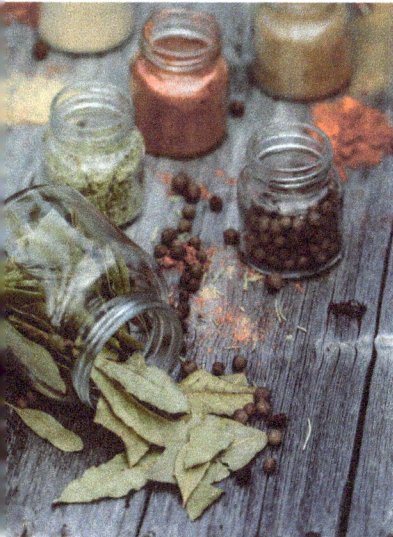

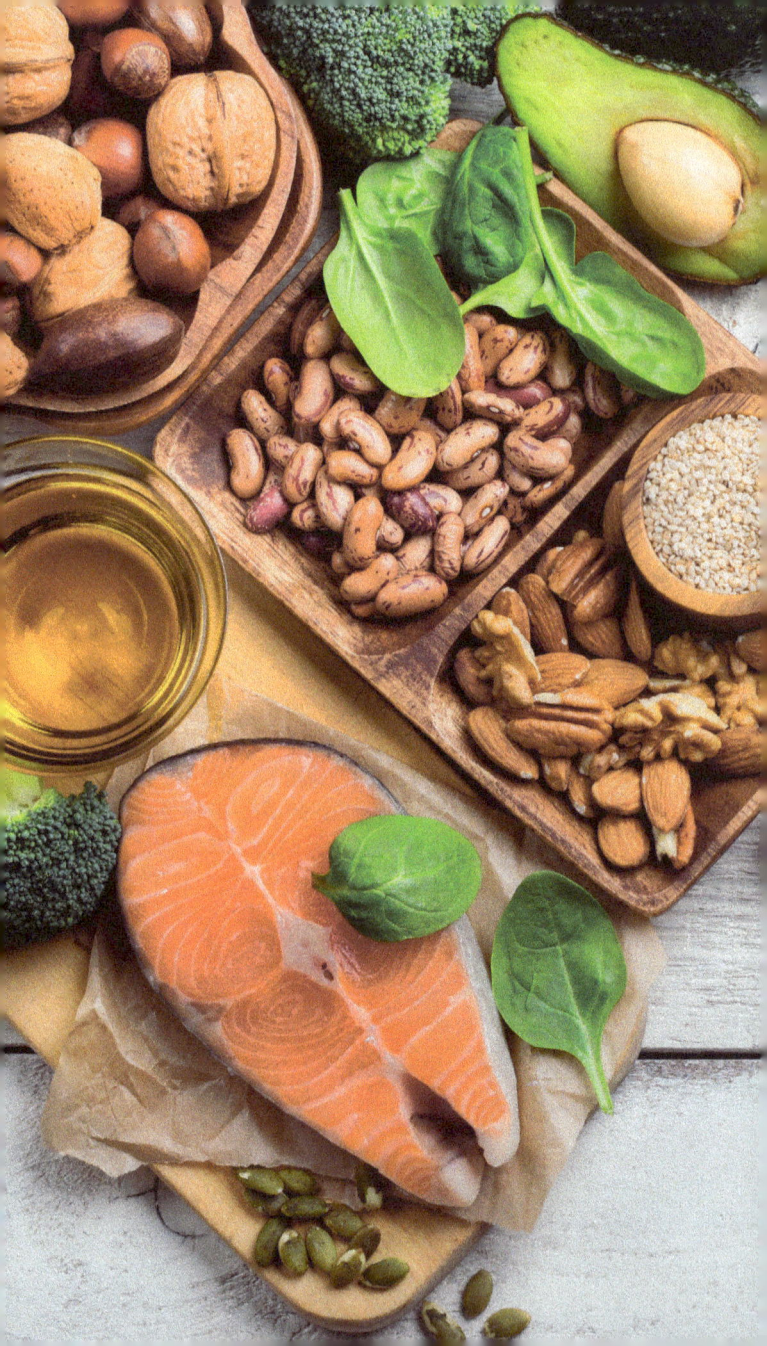

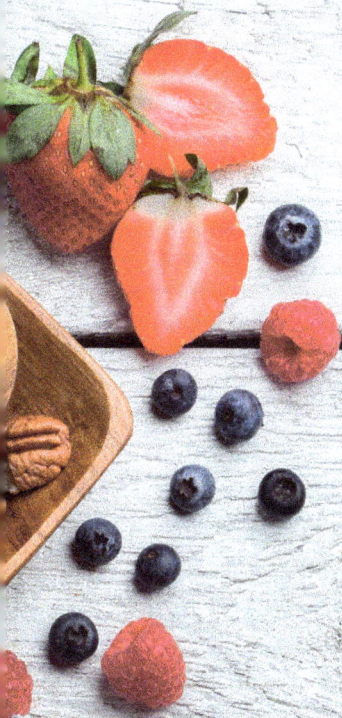

Foods for liver health

Eating the right foods is an important part of any liver cleansing program. It's all very well taking your bespoke herbal formula and diligently flushing, but if you continue to bombard your liver with fatty, indigestible, processed foods, then all of your efforts are going to go to waste.

The following foods are great for supporting your liver health. Like many of the herbs discussed, these foods are bitter in nature and can be incorporated into your daily diet to help improve digestion and overall wellbeing. They should be consumed as part of your liver cleansing program along with fresh seasonal produce that has been lightly cooked and seasoned to make it easily digestible.

Vegetable	Salad	Fruit	Fermented foods	Herbs and spices
Asparagus	Rocket	Bitter melon	Kimchi	Turmeric
Spring greens	Radiccio	Grapefruit	Sauerkraut	Spirulina
Ginger	Horseradish	Rhubarb	Pickled vegetables	Green tea
Samphire	Pak choi	Lemons and limes	Gherkins	Rosemary
Seaweed	Watercress	Cherries	Beetroot	Ginger
Chicory	Garlic	Strawberries		Basil
Artichoke	Chives			Bay leaf
Kale	Salad onions			Cardamom
White cabbage	Pine nuts			Marjoram

Recipes for liver health

Let food be your medicine! The following recipes are quick and easy to put together, and can be adapted in a number of ways to suit your personal taste.

Stock base with bitters

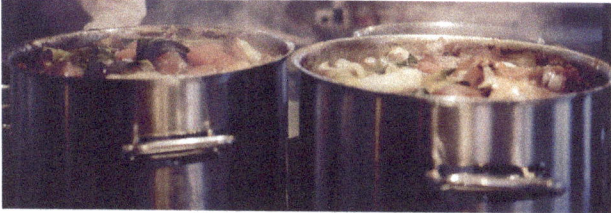

The following recipe is adapted from a wonderful book called 'DIY Bitters' by Guido Masé and Jovial King (see further reading). It's based on the idea of enhancing a base stock which can then be added to soups or stews, along with other bitter herbs and vegetables. This is a fabulously nourishing food to support the health of your microbiome.

Ingredients

- Enough animal bones to fill a litre measuring cup
- 4 medium sized carrots (washed but unpeeled)
- 4 celery stalks
- 1 large onion
- 4 garlic cloves
- 3 x 10 inch (30 cm) burdock roots
- 1 oz (30g) of reishi or shitake mushrooms
- A large bunch of flat leaf parsley
- 4 litres of spring water
- 2 tablespoons of sea salt
- 1 tablespoon of apple cider vinegar
- Grated parmesan cheese to garnish (optional)

Method

Roast the animal bones in an oven for about ten minutes on a low temperature setting. Coarsely chop the vegetables before adding them to a slow cooker or crockpot. Next add the water, sea salt and cider vinegar and throw in the animal bones.

Cover and simmer on a low setting for 8 to 12 hours, adding more water if necessary.

Strain and discard the solids before adding to soups, stews or sauces. The recipe yields about one and a half litres, and so can be frozen in smaller batches for use at a later date.

Spring bitters salad

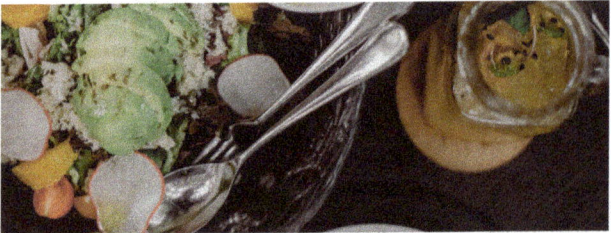

Ingredients

- 1 bunch of dandelion greens coarsely chopped
- A handful of mustard greens coarsely chopped
- Half a fennel bulb, shaved or sliced with a mandolin
- Half a head of red leaf lettuce coarsely chopped
- One cup of mung bean sprouts
- A handful of rocket leaves
- A handful of pumpkin or sunflower seeds

For the dressing

- ¼ of a cup of apple cider vinegar
- ¼ cup of olive oil
- 1 tablespoon of local honey
- ½ teaspoon of oregano
- ½ teaspoon of thyme
- ¼ teaspoon of garlic powder
- 2 teaspoons of wholegrain or Dijon mustard

Method

Prepare the salad leaves by thoroughly washing and then drying with a salad spinner or towel. Combine all the ingredients together in a large glass bowl.

Add the ingredients for the dressing to a small glass jar and whisk with a fork until blended well. The liquid will be of a slightly thicker consistency. Drizzle over your salad and enjoy!

For a more substantial meal, serve with jacket potato, steamed fish or lean, white meat.

Indonesian Jamu Juice –
Turmeric and ginger liver tonic

This bright, marigold coloured drink is an intensely flavoured refreshing tonic made with turmeric, ginger and lime. It is drunk widely across Indonesia for its health benefits, and usually served chilled.

For best results, use fresh turmeric root (although dried can be used if fresh is not available).

Ingredients

- 30g fresh turmeric
- 5g fresh ginger
- 1 - 2 teaspoons of freshly squeezed lime juice
- 1 tablespoon of manuka or local honey
- A small pinch of black pepper
- 250ml of water

Method

Lightly peel the turmeric root to remove any loose skin.

Roughly chop the turmeric and ginger, and add to a food processor or Nutri Bullet along with the water. Remove the resulting liquid from the blender and place in a small glass bowl.

Add boiling water to a saucepan and place the glass bowl containing your Jamu over the top so that it can be gently heated using the *bain marie* method.

Heat the liquid for about 20 minutes or until it has reduced by about half.

Remove from the heat and add the lime juice, honey and pepper.

The Jamu can be drunk hot or allowed to cool and chilled in the fridge.

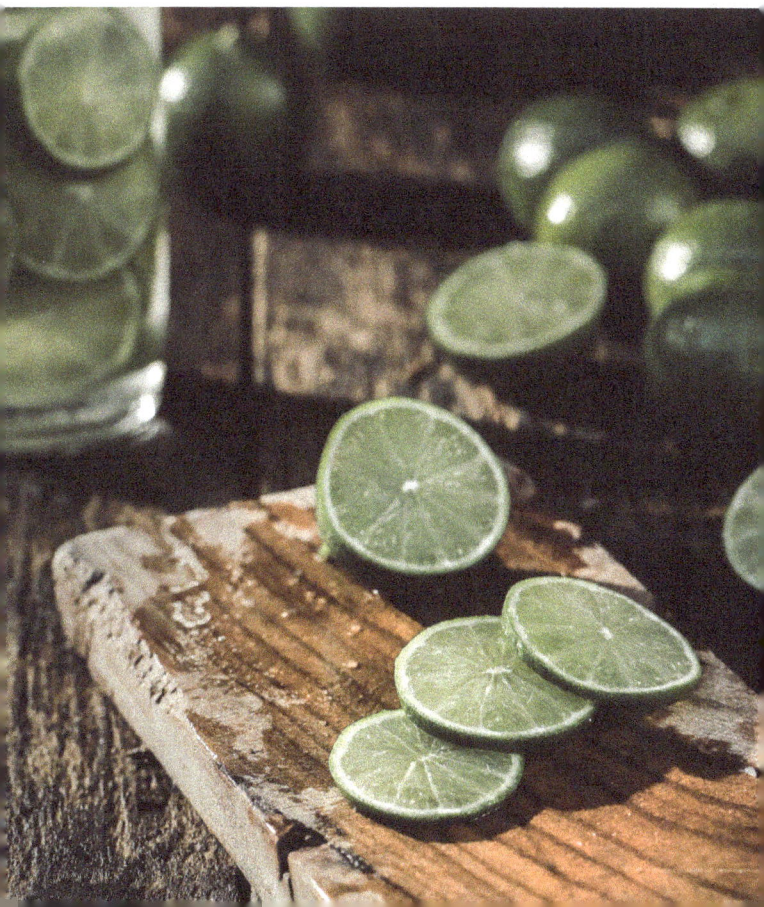

References and further reading

Books

- *The Essential Book of Herbal Medicine* – Simon Mills
- *DIY Bitters* – Guido Masé & Jovial King
- *Healing with Herbs and Foods* – Christopher Hobbs
- *Health through God's Pharmacy* – Maria Treben
- *Make Yourself Better* – Philip Weeks
- *I am Joe's Body - Reader's Digest* – JD Ratcliff
- *Digestive Intelligence - A Holistic View of Your Second Brain* – Irina Matveikova
- *The Amazing Liver Cleanse* – A. Moritz

Website resources, blogs and online articles

Plant monographs from The Herbarium – *https://herbarium.theherbalacademy.com/*

The School of Evolutionary Herbalism Materia Medica – *https://www.evolutionaryherbalism.com/programs*

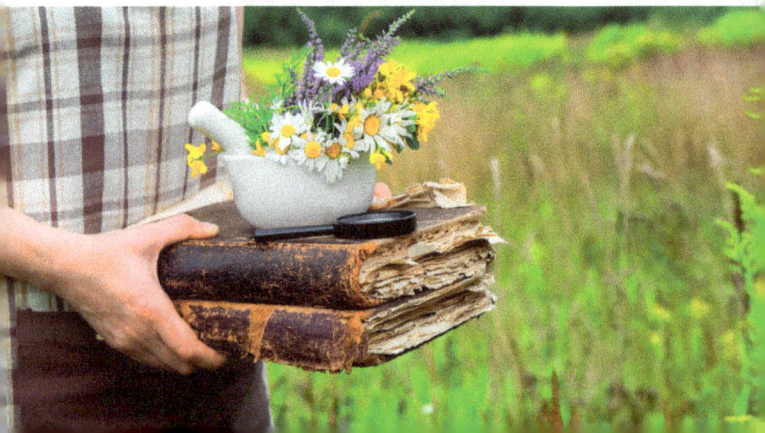

Liver care 101 - Herbs, foods and wellness practices for the liver – *https://theherbalacademy.com/liver-care-101/*

Dark and stormy mushroom bitters – *https://theherbalacademy.com/mushroom-bitters-recipe/*

Alchemilla Apothecary is my own herbal dispensary located on the north Cornwall coast. I stock a range of specialist tinctures (including our high quality range of bitters) as well as offering a bespoke supervised liver detoxification programme.

Swedish bitters is made from a classic blend of 17 different herbs which have been grown within the walls of a Georgian walled kitchen garden. The plants have never been exposed to modern pesticides or herbicides, and the soil is fertilised by natural leaf

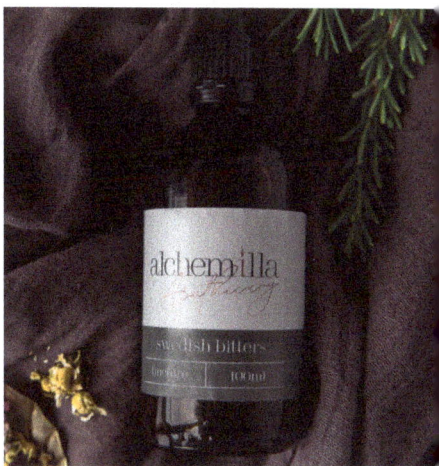

mould collected from the properties own woodland. The product is certified by the British Soil Association.

You can buy Swedish Bitters here – *https://alchemilla.co/herb-store/swedish-bitters/*

Dark and stormy mushroom bitters includes an extract made from lion's mane mushrooms grown locally and hand delivered to the dispensary.

You can buy dark and stormy mushroom bitters here – *https://alchemilla.co/herb-store/dark-stormy-mushroom-bitters/*

Details of my **bespoke liver cleanse programme** can be found here – *https://alchemilla.co/alchemilla-rejuvenate-programme/*

Napiers have been Britain's leading herbal experts since 1860. Run by my supremely knowledgeable colleague Monica Wilde, they stock a wide range of herbal supplies which can be purchased from one of their beautiful, well stocked stores or through their comprehensive website.

G. Baldwin & Co is London's oldest herb shop having first opened its doors in 1844. They sell a wide range of dried herbs and tinctures in small packs for personal use, as well as dispensing to practitioners wishing to place larger wholesale orders. Their customer service is second to none.

About the author

Sarah Murphy is the owner of Alchemilla apothecary, a modern herbal dispensary and integrative wellness clinic located on the beautiful north Cornwall coast.

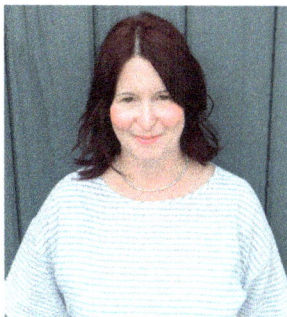

Sarah trained as an herbalist at the College of Naturopathic Medicine in London, and has been in clinical practice for over 12 years. Her special interests lie in the herbal treatment of skin conditions and alternative therapies for supporting people with anxiety and PTSD.

Sarah produces her own range of specialist tinctures manufactured from locally grown plants, and has developed her own skin care range based on the medicinal properties of Kigelia africana (otherwise known as the sausage tree.)

She enjoys collecting and researching traditional recipes from around the world, and has a keen interest in the history of herbal medicine and forgotten plants. She is a member of the Herb Society of Great Britain, and runs regular herb walks and classes on many diverse topics related to herbs and health.

Sarah is a member of the Unified Register of Herbal Practitioners.

You can find out more about her work by visiting her website at *alchemilla.co*

WITH A LOVE FOR BOOKS

With a large range of imprints, from herbalism, selfsufficiency, physical and mental wellbeing, food, memoirs and many more, Herbary Books is shaped by the passion for writing and bringing innovative ideas close to our readers.

All our authors put their hearts into their books and as publishers we just lend a helping hand to bring their creation to life.

Thank you to our authors and to you, dear reader.

Discover and purchase all our books on

WWW.HERBARYBOOKS.COM

HERBARYBOOKS